Aromatherapy for the Soul

Spiritual and Emotional Empowerment with Essential Oils

Judy Jehn, RMT

Vision Publishing, LLC

Denver, CO

1st edition, December 2008

Edited by: Kathryn Caywood

Cover Photography: Judy Jehn

Cover Design: Jeff Eppard

Book Design: Jeff Eppard

International Standard Book Number: ISBN 978-0-9818290-0-5

Library of Congress Control Number: LCCN 2008910276

Jehn, Judy

Aromatherapy for the Soul: Spiritual and Emotional Empowerment with Essential Oils / Judy Jehn.

1. Essential Oils. 2. Aromatherapy. 3. Spiritual life. 4. Soul.

The information provided herein is for educational purposes only and is not intended as a diagnosis, treatment, or prescription for any disease or mental illness. The author, publisher, and distributors accept no responsibility for such use. Those who may be suffering from any disease, illness, or injury should consult with a physician.

Printed in USA

This book is dedicated to all of my teachers who have, are, or will be contributing to my human experience.

PARIS (AP) May 5, 2008- A Roman Catholic bishop said Sunday that the church has officially recognized that the Virgin Mary appeared to a 17th century shepherd girl in the French Alps.

Speaking at Mass in remarks broadcast nationally on France-2 television, Monsignor Jean-Michel di Falco Leandri said he recognized the "supernatural origin" of the apparitions to 17-year-old Benoite Rencurel from 1664 to 1718.

The bishop, in an interview on France-Info radio, said the decision meant the church "has committed itself in an official way to say to pilgrims 'You can come here in total confidence.'" The recognition process involved a panel of experts, including two theologians and an investigating judge, he said.

Officials at Notre-Dame-du-Laus church say that after four months of daily apparitions starting in May 1664, the Virgin Mary asked Rencurel to build a church and a house to receive priests.

The sanctuary, which was founded by Rencurel, today welcomes some 120,000 pilgrims a year—at times providing ***healing oils*** *based on a method that the Virgin Mary was said to pass on to the shepherd girl, the officials said.*

Contents

Chapter 5: Soul Consciousness

Part 2: AromaMethods

Introduction

"You have a brain tumor." His casual manner implied that it was an everyday occurrence. I registered the expression on my brother's face as his eyebrows moved up to the middle of his forehead, but I had no reaction to it myself. The resident continued, "The CAT scan indicates that it is on the left side of your brain, and this explains why you have the paralysis on the right side of your body. If you are going to have a brain tumor, this is the best kind to have. It is called a meningeal tumor, and it is most likely benign."

With that pronouncement and two more hours of waiting and wondering in the emergency room, I was admitted to the hospital; an MRI the following day would disclose more details.

My strong intuition told me that the brain tumor diagnosis was not correct. And, why was the left side of my body also paralyzed?

The severe ache started in my right foot in April, and by August when I went to the emergency room, the immobility and the intense pain (that caused me to cry when I moved) had travelled up my right leg, to my right shoulder and arm, across my back, and down my left side.

The MRI proved me correct. "It's not a brain tumor. It's a tiny spot of scar tissue. I've seen worse on a cadaver!" said the resident. I ignored the cadaver remark; I guessed that he was repeating some quip that might have been an inside joke.

When the chief neurologist entered my room, the energy sizzled with his self-importance. He folded his arms across his chest as his entourage of residents and interns took their positions flanking the end of my bed. With a flick of his hand, he declared that there was nothing physically wrong with me, that my symptoms were all emotional, and that I should follow up with a primary care physician. My counterpoint, that the blood tests indicated that my body was riddled with inflammation, was met with a bemused smile.

The remainder of August and September found me bouncing from one practitioner to another, both alternative and allopathic (western). The answer to my condition was elusive. The pain and the paralysis were linked—of that I was sure. The pain was more intense at times and then would somewhat back off for no apparent reason. Any kind of physical intervention, for instance chiropractic or massage, intensified my reaction and left me agonizingly immobile for days after.

And then, at the end of September, as a friend of mine would say, "God winked." I had the opportunity to travel to the Nova Vita Clinic in Guayaquil, Ecuador. There, under the guidance of D. Gary Young, ND, the founder and president of Young Living Essential Oils, I made the transition from six months of pain and paralysis to wellness in four short weeks.

The trip to Ecuador was one of the bravest journeys of my life. I was alone, in a wheelchair, and did not know what to expect. I just knew that what I was doing was right for me. In hindsight, I also realized that I was embarking on a journey that would change my beingness on many different levels.

Clinic life included an intense routine of exercise, customized diets, daily essential oil supplements and topical applications, IVs, and daily colonics to eliminate the toxicity in my body and give my immune system a chance to rebuild. The therapies varied based on the ongoing assessment of my condition. Initially, I was not able to exercise, but as I began to recover, passive resistance techniques provided the impetus for my mobility. At the clinic and in the patient living quarters, essential oils were being diffused continuously.

I learned that a parasite called cystocercosis was imbedded in my muscles and living off of blood and connective tissue. If left untreated, the possibility that I would be permanently bedridden within two months was very real. The live blood cell analysis shows my condition before and after treatments.

Live Blood Cell Analysis
Judy Jehn

Before
October 15,2007

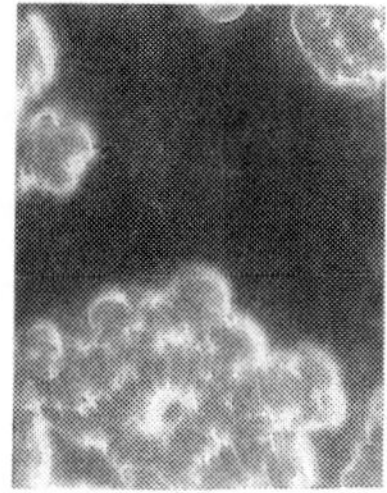

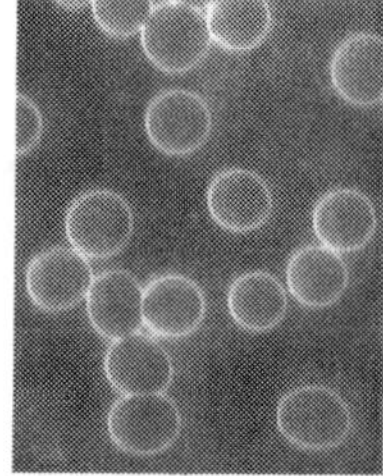

After
November 7,2007

As an independent distributor with Young Living Essential Oils since 1996, I enthusiastically attended lectures by Gary Young. His thought provoking and visionary seminars are always packed with useful essential oil health-related information. In Ecuador, his visits with the patients in the common room became a cherished memory of my clinic experience. He related new plant discoveries, offered sniffs of the newest essential oil distillation, and shared his conversations with the Amazonian Shamans. He also asked our opinions.

Toward the end of my stay, I was healed to the point that I could climb on the back of an ATV. Gary invited the group of patients on a personalized tour of the new Ecuador farm, roughly 2,600 acres, which he was just beginning to cultivate. He devoted nearly six hours of his time as the five of us explored the palo santo glade, the new distillery, and an archeological site on the property. That visit brought mountains of information to me. Gary Young loves what he does, he is extraordinarily good at it, and he is especially generous with his time to help others see his vision.

I respect Gary Young's vision and dedication to build a company that is the world leader of the highest quality, therapeutic grade essential oils. There are other companies that claim to have therapeutic essential oils, but in my opinion, Young Living has the best, most consistent quality, and the most variety.

I left Ecuador with a sense of profound transformation. As I walked through the airports carrying my travel bags, the wheelchair was a distant memory. I knew I was a changed person, but I had no idea how much personal growth and spiritual development I had gone through. I became consciously aware that my life lessons were finally coming into focus. The life-altering experience of being so ill certainly had an impact, but I also gained an intense respect for the emotional and spiritual healing properties of essential oils. I especially value the cumulative beneficial effect of using the oils consistently over time. They have permeated my beingness and have become a new part of me.

This event in my life was an extraordinary journey—finding myself, learning about the beautiful aspects of me, feeling at home in my physical body for the first time, and understanding how and why I am here. I love the result. I love the understanding. I love the emotional connection to my spirit.

My new passion for learning as much as possible about the emotional release and spiritual awareness benefits of essential oils led me to explore new techniques and methods. I practiced first on myself and then solicited willing friends.

As I began to share my revelations and my methodology, people increasingly wanted more information. Then, I awoke one morning to a vision of the cover of this book, including the title and my name as the author. I knew then that I needed to share my journey.

Namaste,
Judy Jehn

Part 1

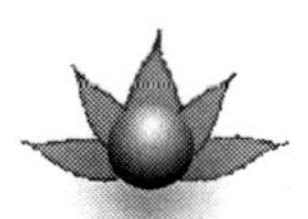

Emotional Awareness and Spiritual Awakening

Chapter 1

The Search for Enlightenment

Pathways to Spirituality

We are all tired of doing the same things over and over again only to get the same result, when all we want is for our life to change.

Many techniques are already available and thousands of books have been written on the vast subject of releasing emotional patterns, changing our lives, and the Law of Attraction. The focus varies but the message is the same. The "I think, therefore I am" mentality is catching on all over, and everyone wants a quick cure because we are learning as never before that meditation and affirmations are magic bullets.

But changing our lives involves more than just positive thoughts and go-for-the-gold manifestations. There is an acceptance of the human body as an energetic entity. The body's vibrational frequency either rejects or propels other energies, changing the human existence into different states of being. So the next wave of self-help books includes these energy healing concepts, as well as spirituality, or the connection to the soul. Authors are sending explicit messages about how to find our spiritual path and how to change our vibrational frequency to manifest what we want in life.

The premise of this book is that both the life force energy and the fragrance of pure, unadulterated essential oils enhance emotional release and spiritual awakening. Powerful plant essences encourage our progress toward spiritual growth by accessing the emotional area of the brain and permitting the release of pent-up feelings.

Balancing the body's energy through the use of essential oils creates a sense of inner peace and harmony that lets the soul open to the most grandeur possible. The oils of life from the plants of the earth are synergistic with the spiritual processes.

With inhalation, the essential oils carry fragrant molecules to the brain stimulating emotional release. When super-oxygenating molecules penetrate the brain with phytonutrients beneficial to the cells, we have the best possible combination of positive energy and positive emotional balance.

Spirituality is hard to define because it is personal and individual. It could be a religion, a belief system, a way of life, meditation, prayer, music, or any other means to connect to your soul. I think of spirituality as my link to my inner strength through my Higher Source, which I call God. You may have another name like Divinity, Spirituality, Universe, Higher Consciousness, Buddha or whatever name that you choose. This book uses the term *Higher Source* to denote that spiritual beingness. The conscious revelation is distributed equally to every incarnated being as we choose to tune into, accept, and absorb the Higher Source within us.

The change in beingness seems difficult for some and easy for others. The important concept is to honor it, believe in it, and to trust the process.

We are spiritual beings inhabiting human bodies, rather than human beings with a spirit. Once we evolve past humanness and recognize the *spiritualness* of our human existence, our perspective changes. When we do that, we are altered beings, both here on planet earth and in the intergalactic systems that create our universe.

Letting Go of the Past

As spiritual beings, physical existence is a means of continuing the soul's growth. Recognizing that we are here to further our spiritual journey, our human form is a creation that we chose in order to help the spirit along its road toward fulfillment.

No one has the right to tell us how to proceed on our spiritual path. We alone have the responsibility for our soul's choice, to know at a soul level the chosen direction that we are to follow.

The challenges are ours alone. Understanding and smoothing out the roller-coaster of feelings is like a giant first step.

Consider that there is constant opportunity for emotional re-programming. When you have an experience similar to one in the past, you do not need to expect the same result. As you let go of your past, your behavioral responses to certain stimuli changes.

Think of your body as a bio-computer. When you add a program to your computer, it must be installed in the proper sequence. The installation process accesses the hard drive and places all of the subprograms in the appropriate places for the software to execute.

Similarly, when you want to remove a piece of software, you perform a de-installation process. This removes all of the subprograms that were added during the installation.

Now apply the same concept to the emotional body. Your emotions begin their programming from birth. And over your entire lifetime, your emotional responses are constantly being reinforced. This hard-wired emotional software causes physiological reactions in response to your emotional events.

Just as in the computer example, emotional programming cannot simply be deleted. Re-programming appears to be the most effective means for changing behavioral responses by honoring, accepting, and then letting go of the emotion. Alternative behaviors, or constructive new reactions to the feelings, installs new emotional software, aids in the shift, and helps to attain the sought after new patterns. Part 2 of this book includes techniques using essential oils that assist in developing constructive new behaviors.

How do we acquire our emotional blueprint? From very early childhood, our know-how is defined for us. We notice the reactions of others, learning from example how to feel and to act in response to certain stimuli. And if we do not behave in the way that we are supposed to, we are cajoled, punished, ignored, abused, manipulated, even ridiculed until the reactive pattern is formed.

Is this the real person? Or is this the programming that we accepted because of conformity, societal norms, family habits, religious beliefs, or Miss Manners' protocols? We grew up with these past feelings forming an unconscious life pattern. This is our emotional software that is running all of the time.

We become hard-wired, using the same emotional guidebook over and over again. We try to change, but we still respond the same way to the stimuli and encounter the same outcome. This leads to frustration, and eventually we give up.

We all know someone who repeatedly complains about their situation or a negative experience. They are defining themselves in the past by using their emotional guidebook. They do not have a basis for identifying themselves in the present, much less seeing their future possibilities.

The healing only happens when you are in present time—when you have the presence to recognize that you are able to let go, that you are able to trust, and that you can disconnect from what does not feel right anymore. Present time means reacting in the moment, no longer dwelling in the past, and no longer projecting the dysfunction into the future.

Understanding that your past does not control your adult decision making is a giant leap toward the healing process, and is the chance for the eventual fulfillment of your goals and desires. When you are in present time, the past no longer defines you.

"Get over it" sounds too simple to most of us who have a history of some kind of abuse, but dwelling on that abuse and labeling ourselves a victim only serves as an excuse to keep from moving forward. What is important is the knowledge that we no longer need to be a product of our past—we are only responsible for who we have become in the present.

The life force energy of essential oils acts as a catalyst to bring us into the present time, bringing the changes that we so desire. We now have an alternative that may lead us to emotional freedom.

It's Just Energy!

Each of us has an energy field—actually energy layers—representing body, mind, and spirit. This energy field extends outward and communicates our inner state of being. In fact, we are walking billboards advertising our mental-emotional state to the world. Most people can sense this in others, but we are all capable of tuning into our higher senses, and this helps us to understand more about ourselves and others. (Chapter 5 covers this in detail.) The energy that we see, feel, and hear is our mirror, which is translated by our emotions through our energy field complex. It determines how we experience and respond to an interaction with another person.

When we experience a negative emotion, we are literally declaring that feeling in our energy field, and others subliminally sense and respond to it.

Suppose that you feel slighted by not being included in a conversation at work. Your emotional energy around that feeling is in your energy field and is picked up by others. Your co-worker may choose to keep away from you in order to avoid a confrontation. But, you expected this reaction because this is one of your patterns that repeat over and over again.

The key to changing the outcome is to change the energy. By understanding the principles of the energy entity, also called the energy body, and how the interconnectedness of the emotional and physical body manifests the energy body outcome, we most assuredly have the capability to affect our wishes and wants. Integration of our innermost aspirations and desired results is fulfilled when the entire blueprint of our body, mind, and spirit is in alignment. (Chapters 3 and 4 cover Emotional Energy and Life Force Energy, respectively.)

Alternative energetic healing techniques, all claiming successes in clearing the body's energy field, are proliferating at this time. Some of these healing methods include Reiki, Yuen Method, Matrix Energetics, Emotional Freedom Technique (EFT), and Spiritual Response Technique (SRT). This is only a sampling; there are many more. The intention of these therapies is to clear negative energy, shift it into a more positive state, balance the polarity, or all of the above. In any given circumstance, it can be difficult to determine the right modality for yourself. Practitioners vary in experience from well-trained professionals to novices who hang up a shingle after a three day weekend workshop.

No matter the method used, adding essential oils to any healing modality generates more room for expansion, the opportunity to move ahead, to open up, and to reach even further into our understanding of the conscious and the unconscious, the spiritual, and the physical. This allows the physical body to shift, the emotional body to release unwanted patterns, and the spiritual soul to awaken from within.

As a massage therapist, I know that using essential oils helps to assuage the physical aches and pains that bring my clients to me, but it also opens up avenues for them to grow and develop personally, mentally, and emotionally. I see it happen. I observe their progress. I delight in their well-being.

My clients come to me because they claim that I give the best massages, but I know that the essential oils are a significant part of their experience. In addition to massage, adding essential oils when performing Reiki or other energy healing techniques magnifies the benefits of all my healing methods and produces longer lasting and more positive effects in my clients.

The synergy of incorporating essential oils with natural healing techniques will continue to be the subject of future research papers. My intention in this book is to share what I have been taught and what I have learned intuitively through my own personal experiences with my emotional and physical healing using the oils.

Transformation

We are moving toward a more enlightened view and science is only now beginning to discover new pathways to the unconscious mind. According to the quantum physicists, astrologers, and spiritual healers or light workers, the life forces on the planet are shifting and moving with increasing speed.

This new consciousness teaches us that we are advancing metaphysically. We live in a time of vast re-alignment, spiritual growth, and emotional healing on many levels.

If we think back on the lives that our parents and grandparents lived, we glimpse the marked differences to where we are today. Can you imagine your parents or grandparents talking about essential oils, auras, chakras and energy centers, or releasing emotional patterns? And yet it is somewhat common today. Even if people do not believe in the concepts or their implication, most have at least heard the terminology.

We have the power to transform our lives. People are doing it. Making positive change enhances self-confidence. Confidence promotes self-esteem and allows for the release of ego. The process continues until you are personally aware that you have really made a difference. It becomes a positive Catch-22!

Essential oils are the power behind trusting your new instincts, letting go, and disconnecting from what does not seem self-supportive anymore. The essential oils enhance our new associations that allow us to be in alignment with our souls, our true and authentic selves. The oils really are miraculous in this respect!

Each essential oil has its own set of characteristics. I like to think of them as having their own personalities, which helps to bring things back to a human scale. Not everyone will use the same oils to achieve their desired result. Each of us will be attracted to different essential oils because each of us is different and has a unique set of circumstances.

There is no greater teacher than essential oils. Learn to trust them and trust the healing effect that they provide throughout your entire body. As you begin to experience the curative properties of essential oils, your intuition becomes more powerful and your awareness grows.

And then, most wonderfully, use the life force energy of essential oils to support and enhance your body through spiritual and emotional growth to reach the desired state of development and sanguinity.

Chapter 2

The Power of Essential Oils

Aromatherapy and Essential Oils

The terms *aromatherapy* and *essential oils* are generally used interchangeably these days. *Aromatherapy* originally referred to the use of highly fragrant, pure, medicinal grade plant essential oils used for restorative health benefits and for unlocking the emotions. The name *aromatherapy* is currently so widely used that its meaning has been reduced to include synthetically scented lotions, potions, candles, and plug-ins which have no therapeutic value and can actually be harmful to humans.

The reintroduction of aromatherapy and essential oils into modern medicine began in the early 1900's with the work of the French cosmetic chemist René-Maurice Gattefossé, PhD. He and a group of scientists began studying plant essences in 1907, and he is generally deemed the father of aromatherapy, as he coined the term in 1928. A very similar term, *aroma-terii*, was used in the 15th century to designate the importance of aromatic plant extracts and essential oils that were used in the apothecaries of that time.

Ancient Uses

The history of essential oils dates back to at least 4,500 BC and the ancient Egyptians, who had become skilled in the process of extracting plant essences. They used oils and other plant aromatics for religious rituals, the treatment of illness, and other physical and spiritual needs. In everyday life, the Egyptians used fragrances for personal scents, ceremonies in the temples, rituals in the pyramids, embalming, and for medicinal purposes.

Hieroglyphics found on the walls of Egyptian temples describe hundreds of oil recipes and how to blend the various single oils for physical and emotional benefits. Researchers believe that a sacred room in the Temple of Isis, on the island of Philae, depicts the Cleansing the Flesh and Blood of Evil Deities, an emotional clearing ritual that required three days of cleansing using essential oils. Other temples provide information on medicinal formulas that were used by the high priests.

The Egyptians stored their sacred oils in elaborately decorated alabaster jars sealed with beeswax. Specially designed evaporation dishes were used in the temples to diffuse fragrance for religious rituals.

When King Tut's tomb was opened in 1922, many alabaster jars were found. It is said the jars once held a total of 350 liters of essential oils and that some of the jars still contained traces of oils on what remained of the waxy seals. Researchers believe that tomb robbers stole nearly all of the essential oils, but left the gold and jewelry behind. This indicates how valuable the fragrant oils were to this ancient civilization.

Other civilizations also used aromatic plant oils. The Hebrews learned from the Egyptians and documented their recipes in the Torah. The many applications of fragrance became a hallmark of the Roman Empire, where people were avid users of essential oils to purify their temples and enhance their baths. In the 10th century, the Arabians discovered a method of distillation that allowed for more efficient extraction of essential oils from the plants. Similar forms of that distillation method are in use today.

One of the oldest known medical records is the Ebers Papyrus, a scroll over 870 feet long that was written in hieroglyphics and dates from the 16th century BC. Found in Egypt in the 1870s, it contains remedies, prescriptions, and recipes for the diagnosis and treatment for over 800 ailments and injuries.

Gold, Frankincense, and Myrrh

Essential oils played an important role in the lives of biblical people. In the ancient world, essential oils were considered more valuable than gold. For example, Moses used them to protect the Israelites from disease, and Mary and Joseph used them to keep baby Jesus and themselves healthy.

The Bible contains over 500 references to oils for healing, cleansing, and holy anointing. The 12 essential oils most frequently mentioned in the Bible include **aloes (sandalwood), cassia, cedarwood, cypress, frankincense, galbanum, hyssop, myrrh, myrtle, onycha, cistus (rose of Sharon), and spikenard.**

Frankincense may have been the most important oil in ancient times. It was revered by royalty and used to anoint kings, especially the newborn children of the kings' lineage. This essential oil was distilled from the resin harvested from the **frankincense** tree. The resin was considered so precious that any laborer caught stealing it was subject to severe penalty, which included having their hand chopped off or loss of life for a subsequent offense.

To this day, the Catholic Church uses **frankincense** in the incense form for its ceremonies. Did the early Church Fathers know that burning the incense could help ward off disease, infections, and other spiritually negative elements? It is very possible! It is also possible that the early Catholic

Church recognized that **frankincense** enhanced prayer and meditation. Today, science has proved that the molecules of **frankincense** essential oil pass through the blood-brain barrier and stimulate the pineal and pituitary glands—an action that may encourage meditative or prayer consciousness.

Myrrh was used in a variety of ways because of its anti-infectious properties. The ancient Egyptians embalmed their mummies with **myrrh** because of its effectiveness in preventing bacterial growth. Greek soldiers nursed their battle wounds with **myrrh** essential oil. Expectant mothers used **myrrh** to ward off infection and to elevate their moods. The Ebers Papyrus contains many recipes using **myrrh** essential oil and honey. Today, **myrrh** is used for its ability to help with skin and throat infections, and regeneration of skin tissue.

Modern Day Discovery

In his 1937 book, Dr. Gattefossé told the story of his discovery of the incredible properties of **lavender** essential oil. As a result of a laboratory accident in 1910, his hands were covered with a rapidly developing gas gangrene. He reportedly plunged his hands into a beaker of **lavender** essential oil, which stopped the gasification of the tissue. Due to the amazing restorative properties of the pure **lavender** essential oil, Dr. Gattefossé's hands healed quickly and with little scarring.

During World War II, Dr. Jean Valnet, MD, a colleague of Dr. Gattefossé, began using therapeutic-grade essential oils on patients suffering from battlefield injuries when he ran out of antibiotics. This became one of the first modern, live research experiments in understanding the powerful effect of essential oils to combat and counteract infection. With essential oils, he was able to save the lives of many soldiers who might otherwise have died.

Two of Dr. Valnet's students, Dr. Paul Belaiche, MD and Dr. Jean-Claude Lapraz, MD, expanded his work through the clinical investigation of the antiviral, antibacterial, antifungal, and antiseptic properties in essential oils. Because of the work of these doctors and scientists, the field of essential oils and aromatherapy has become a burgeoning industry. Dr. Daniel Pénoël, MD, is considered the modern day French champion of essential oils.

I believe that D. Gary Young, the founder and president of Young Living Essential Oils, is the most knowledgeable person on the planet regarding the use of medicinal grade essential oils for everyday use. His expertise extends to plant culture, growth, harvesting, and distillation to create the best therapeutic value from the plants.

Learning From the Plant Kingdom

Essential oils are complex, highly concentrated natural plant substances commonly referred to as the life force, blood, or vital fluid of the plant. These liquids are called volatile, meaning that they easily evaporate, and are stored in the plant stems, roots, leaves, flowers, or bark. Essential oils are used during the plant's life cycle to transport nutrients to the cells, thus allowing the plant to grow, develop, and adapt to its surroundings. When a plant is cut or the exterior is damaged in some way, the liquid that bleeds out and seals the injured area is the essential oil.

When you inhale a plant's fragrance, the distinct aroma is the plant's essential oil. That is why rose smells different than rosemary or lemon smells different from lemongrass.

This fragrance is what plants use to communicate. Plants release their volatile fluids atmospherically. Their aroma actually serves the plant by attracting humans and animals with the appeal of its fragrances and flavors or by attracting pollinators. Some plants mutually stimulate each others growth, while other plants use aroma for defense by repelling other plants, insects, and animals. Many organic farmers apply this knowledge in the way they group plants together using a technique called *companion planting* or *agrophytocoenosis*.

The Science of Aromatherapy

All essential oils have a unique compatibility with the organs and tissue of the human body. The oils contain chemical constituents that are molecularly bioavailable and act synergistically with the body's biochemical functions. They are comprised of amino acids, which are the building blocks of every cell. This unique compatibility with human protein enables them to be readily identified and accepted by human organs and tissues. Essential oils distribute oxygen, amino acids, enzymes, and other nutrients throughout the tissue. In the body, they metabolize within two to three hours and do not accumulate in the tissue, as opposed to synthetic medicines that can build up in the liver, kidneys, colon, and other organs.

Science recognizes over 70,000 different kinds of aromatic molecules in plants. The uniqueness of each different essential oil and the effect on the human body becomes the basis for the science of aromatherapy. Over 300 different essential oils are being distilled or extracted today, and each single essential oil has a unique set of chemical properties.

The original French medical texts tell us that essential oils can be antibacterial, antifungal, anti-infectious, anti-inflammatory, immune enhancing, and much more. For example, these texts say that **frankincense** is antitumoral and immunostimulating, **cypress** helps to increase circulation, and **oregano** and **thyme** are highly antiviral.

The National Library of Medicine has over 4,000 research articles on essential oils and the list is growing. Documented evidence demonstrates that compounds in some essential oils destroy drug-resistant cancer cells. Current studies show that essential oils are highly effective against antibiotic resistant super bugs—for example, MRSA, which stands for *methicillin resistant staphylococcus aureus*.

Essential Oils have a wide variety of uses. For example, **oregano** and **thyme** have the ability to clear the receptor sites of hormone cells that are blocked by petrochemicals. The antioxidant power of **clove** oil is unparalleled in the prevention of cell mutation and as a free radical scavenger.

The vast array of potential uses for essential oils includes personal use in pain relief, massage, skin care, hair care, and oral health care. They are used on animals and humans from infants to the elderly. They clean wounds, control the bleeding, eradicate infection, reduce congestion, stop viruses, soothe nerves, calm inflammation, relax muscles, and bring on a sense of well-being. The list is endless.

As a word of caution, most essential oils sold in retail stores and on the internet are perfume or cosmetic grade and cannot be effectively used medicinally. Many oils are diluted with linalyl acetate, propylene glycol, or alcohols to speed up the distillation process and stretch the product, making the oils less expensive for the retail consumer. Adulterated oils may cause harm to the human body through the absorption of petrochemicals and synthetics.

It is estimated that only 2 percent of all of the essential oils that are produced in the world are therapeutic grade and used for medicinal purposes; the rest are targeted for commercial use and end up in fragrances and even food.

D. Gary Young is a current-day David challenging the Goliath of adulterated oils that are sold and labeled as "100% pure."

The intended purpose of pure essential oils is for sustaining the physical, mental, emotional, and spiritual bodies of our humanness and balancing homeostasis. They penetrate cell membranes, transport oxygen and nutrients to the blood and tissues, stimulate cellular regeneration, and enhance electrical frequencies. They are electrically alive and studies evidence the ability of essential oils to repair or erase faulty genetic coding and restore the natural frequency of the cells.

Essential oils are beautifully complex, concentrated, powerful, and yet simple. Just a drop or two of the right therapeutic grade essential oil can produce immediate and pronounced results.

Not only are essential oils the life blood of the plant, but they are highly beneficial to humans. From the physical realm to the emotional and spiritual, they have properties that soothe the senses, invigorate the body, and promote well-being.

Chapter 3

The Force of Emotions

Emotions and the Sense of Smell

Our sense of smell triggers our emotions, which can bring about positive or negative reactions. When we think of aromatherapy, we are naturally attracted to uplifting, rejuvenating, or relaxing scents.

Essential oil fragrances are being explored through a relatively new science called *olfactotherapy* or *olfactology* because of the potential restorative properties of smell on the emotions. Research shows that as a fragrance is inhaled, the sense of smell exerts strong influence on the hypothalamus, considered the hormone command center, and the limbic portion of the brain, which is the seat of the emotions.

We smell with our brain. The body-mind interpretation of smell results from the frequency, shape, and size of the molecules. Researchers have long held that we interpret scent by the shape of airborne molecules. However, more recent scientific studies now suggest that we smell based on the vibration theory, the process by which the body distinguishes one odor molecule from another by its energy, the way it vibrates. It is now believed that vibration triggers smell recognition, and the molecular shape and size determine the intensity. The multi-billion dollar perfume industry is exploiting this information.

Our sense of smell is amazingly complex and beautifully created. We have two nostrils and two olfactory bulbs, and through some very elaborate physiology, we interpret or distinguish from 10,000 to 100,000 different odors via an estimated 800,000 nerve receptors. This is 10 to 100 times more receptors than we have for sight or hearing.

The olfactory receptors, about the size of a postage stamp, occupy an area in the roof of each nasal cavity. Air entering the nasal cavities makes a hairpin turn when entering the respiratory passage way, so sniffing or deep breathing intensifies the sense of smell because more air flows across the olfactory receptors.

Scent goes directly to the receptor sites in the olfactory membrane, which transmits the aroma to the amygdala gland in the emotional center of the brain. The amygdala gland sits in the temporal lobe centered between the two cerebral hemispheres. It is a small almond shaped neural structure, and it plays a role in the sense of smell, motivation, and emotion.

The neural anatomy of the limbic part of the brain responds only to smell. It does not understand spoken or written words. Our other senses are wired differently in the cerebral lobes. The amygdala, with its extraordinary function of emotional processing using sensory information, suggests that a direct pathway to bring about conscious and unconscious positive emotional conditioning is through the sense of smell.

Memories are not actually stored in the limbic–emotional part of the brain. It is believed that the amygdala manages the storage and filing system for all of our emotional experiences. The body is composed of an estimated 60 to 100 trillion cells, and within each cell there are DNA strands of additional memory. This giant body bio-computer becomes the repository for our emotions, and the limbic brain directs the placement and retrieval of those memories.

Smell triggers memories. We have all experienced the familiar chocolate chip cookie smell and the sense of comfort and joy that it brings. How about the perfume, now old-fashioned, that floods you with memories of your mother? Or the delicious-smelling pasta dish that takes you back to your trip to Italy? Or the ball glove smells that brings up the days of playing catch with your dad? Smell can suggest other memories as well. Hospital smells, school smells, nursing home smells, pollution smells, or smoke smells. Smell can evoke a memory or an incident from your past that you had not thought of in years.

Our emotional experiences are the source for our memories. Theorists believe that many of these memories may occur on an unconscious level and become the basis for our emotional behavior patterns.

Psychotherapy and hypnotherapy support the idea of brain self-control, which means doing something that provokes a positive emotional reaction in the brain. This consciously unlocks the emotions at an unconscious level, whereas the alternative modalities of meditation and affirmations work to alter the neuro-functioning at the conscious level.

Conscious control of this neurobiological function through positive olfactory stimulation with essential oils, together with reinforcement, may have significant and profound effects on releasing emotional patterns.

Emotional Energy

Electrically charged feelings are the energy of emotion. Writers often refer to emotions as being energy in motion. Many believe that negative emotions are considered to resonate at lower frequencies, while positive emotions vibrate at higher levels. Therapeutic grade oils are emotionally compatible because the essential oil molecules vibrate at frequencies that are equal to or higher than those found in the human body. Applying an essential oil with a higher electromagnetic charge raises a negative emotional vibration.

How do emotional energies influence us and those around us? You can always tell when a confident, successful person enters the room because they resonate with accomplishment, power, and achievement. Their appearance or what they say seems to be of less importance than simply their stature. You can actually feel their energy. Their self-presence is an indication that their goals and objectives are in alignment with their emotions. That powerful magnetic force is frequently referred to as their energetic body, energy field, aura, or etheric field. While the terms vary slightly in meaning, they are generally used interchangeably. The energy body is simultaneously and inexorably linked to the physical and the emotional state of the person.

Everything in life is energy, from the humblest amoeba to giant sequoias. It is all a matter of frequency, the speed of the vibration. Every cell, organ, and system in our body vibrates at a specific frequency, as do our feelings and emotions.

Our emotions become a physical force in our energy field. An example would be how we know if someone is ecstatic or angry, even without that person having to verbalize the feeling, by noticing their body language. We feel the energy about them. We even have words that seemingly correspond to the resonant frequency that we feel, for example vibrant, elated, joyous, sad, depressed, or unhappy.

We actively interact with frequencies all the time. Sound has frequency, as do color and light. As we experience the ebb and flow of frequency, different energies push against us, and this is reflected in our moods, emotions, and even our physical bodies. When listening to upbeat, happy music we have the urge to dance, while the music at a funeral is consistent with the somber mood of the grieving friends and family. On the Fourth of July, the light and color energy of the fireworks are timed with the beat of the music, creating a patriotic feeling. The frequency of emotions is real and normal.

Emotions move and flow in our reality with ups and downs as predictable and unpredictable mood swings. In actuality, these mood swings are really energy in motion and reflect changes in the physical, emotional, and energetic bodies. As an example, why does a person suddenly have road rage when they seemed perfectly normal the moment before? Think about what happens when a person looks at their lottery ticket and registers that they have just won the grand prize?

Emotions share energy with physical body parts. Positive (constructive) or negative (destructive) emotions have signature frequencies and are linked to associated physical manifestations or dysfunctions. Research has been conducted on the relationship between feelings and disease, and books by Louise L. Hay (*Heal Your Body*), and Karol K. Truman (*Feelings Buried Alive Never Die...*), elaborate on the importance of emotional well-being in order to obtain optimal health, functioning, and balance.

In order to understand why essential oils are so effective in the area of vibrational energy, it is valuable to have some scientific background on frequency. Frequency is defined as the measurable rate of electrical energy flow between two points. According to the late Dr. Royal R. Rife, healthy humans resonate at a frequency of between 62 and 78 megahertz (MHz). Using a frequency generator that he developed and experimented with from the early 1920s to the late 1930s, Dr. Rife concluded that every disease could also be measured, and that the frequency of disease was lower than the optimal resonating frequency of the human body. His practice showed that a substance with a higher frequency could destroy a disease with a lower frequency. For example, we know that laughter raises our bodily frequency.

While Dr. Rife's work was considered highly controversial at the time, this research has a cult following, with scientists pursuing this area of interest today. Commonly held frequencies are represented in the table below:

Frequency and the Human Body

Human Brain	72-90 MHz
Human Body	62-68 MHz
Cold Symptoms	58 MHz
Flu Symptoms	57 MHz
Candida	55 MHz
Epstein Barr	52 MHz
Cancer	42 MHz
Death begins	25 MHz

Foods

Processed/canned food	0 MHz
Fresh Produce	up to 15 MHz
Dry Herbs	12-22 MHz
Fresh Herbs	20-27 MHz

Further research reveals that negative thoughts may lower the body's frequency by as much as 12 MHz, while positive thoughts are similarly able to raise the body's frequency by up to 10 MHz. Prayer and meditation are said to powerfully increase frequency by 15 MHz.

By comparison, therapeutic grade essential oils range between 52 MHz to as high as 320 MHz, which is the frequency of therapeutic grade rose oil.

Following Dr. Rife's conclusions, some experts agree that the application of therapeutic oils can encourage the cells to resonate at higher frequencies, providing the body with an opportunity to restore homeostasis. Therapeutic grade oils change the genetic structuring by calming the central nervous system through the amygdala and pineal gland, and thus enabling the release of stored up trauma and negative emotions.

Lower frequencies are associated with the physical body, middle range frequencies relate to emotional well-being, and higher frequencies are associated with spiritual consciousness. Raising the body's natural frequency through the use of therapeutic grade essential oils helps to release emotional blockages and increase spiritual empowerment.

Inhaling Essential Oils for Emotional Balance

Through the sense of smell essential oils present a remarkable opportunity for healing emotions. We choose oils for physical healing and also for emotional balance, along with anti-stress or mood-stabilizing effects. We have an affinity for fragrances that are actually good for us, so we can rely on our noses and our instincts for choosing oils beneficial to us. Although the aroma of some oils may not be appealing to us, interestingly those are perhaps the ones most needed for releasing the emotional patterns.

Here are a number of ways to inhale essential oils to influence the emotional brain:

Direct Inhalation

- Inhale directly from the bottle. Start with the open bottle at your navel, bringing it slowly up to about an inch from your nose. Inhale evenly as you do this. Slowly wave the bottle under your nostrils while breathing deeply. With your right fingers, close your right nostril and inhale from the left. Do the same from the opposite side. Return to breathing the aroma from both nostrils. The technique of breathing through your left nostril first is intended to initially stimulate the right or creative side of the brain, before the logic, or left, portion of the brain.

- Place two or more drops into the palm of your left hand and rub clockwise with the flat palm of your right hand. Cup your hands together over your nose and mouth and inhale deeply. (Be careful not touch your eyes! If essential oil gets into your eyes, do not use water. Dilute with a vegetable oil.)

- Add several drops of an essential oil to a bowl of hot, but not boiling, water and inhale the vapors that rise from the bowl. To increase the intensity of the oil vapors, drape a towel over your head and bowl while breathing in the vapors.

Indirect or Subtle Inhalation

- Choose the same places that you would ordinarily apply perfume and put a drop or several drops on your chest, neck, upper sternum, wrists, under your nose, and behind your ears. Breathe in the fragrance throughout the day.
- Wear a clay diffuser as a necklace scented with your favorite essential oil.
- Apply oils to a cotton ball, tissue, or handkerchief and place it on the heating and air conditioning vents in your house or on the air vent of your car. Use natural fabrics rather than synthetic.

Diffusing

- Diffusing creates a pleasant environment for inhalation in addition to reducing airborne bacteria, fungus, mold and unpleasant odors. A variety of diffusers are available, including aromatic mist, fan, nebulizing, plug-in, and ultra-sonic.
- They are designed to atomize a micro-fine mist of essential oils into the air so the mist can remain in suspension for several hours. Most diffusers have a mist regulator that helps to control the amount of oil used. Appliance timers are helpful for regulating diffusing times, which are typically five to 15 minutes per hour for creating an aromatic environment.
- Heating or burning essential oils (such as candles or burners) reduces the beneficial therapeutic effects and could even create toxic compounds.

Essential Oils for Positive Feelings

Essential oil aromas affect our emotions in ways that cannot be accessed by any other means. Buried emotions can create discordant patterns. Here are some essential oils and oil blends to elevate the mood and soothe the psyche.

Bonding – **Purification**

Choice Making – **Purification, palo santo**

Contentment – **Evergreen Essence**

Harmony – **Harmony**

Happiness – **Joy, Highest Potential**

Inner Balance – **Inner Child, Present Time, Release**

Inner Direction – **spruce, Envision, Highest Potential, Inspiration, Motivation, Surrender, Valor**

Internalization – **Believe, Inner Child**

Letting Go - **Forgiveness, Release**

Manifestation - **Transformation**

Reflection – **Joy**

Self Worth – **frankincense, cedarwood, palo santo, myrrh**

Spirit – **Christmas Spirit**

Transformation – **Transformation**

Unconditional Love – **myrrh**

Chapter 4

Life Force Energy

The Spiritual Energy Centers of the Soul

There is a tendency to look outside ourselves to find spirituality. However, spirituality comes from within because the body is really the temple for the soul.

Synagogues, temples, churches, and other highly energized and spiritually evocative earth sites are marvelous locations for peace and respite, and I am awed every time I enter a beautiful place of worship or visit a natural area. But you do not need to physically be in a sacred place to access your Higher Source.

Quantum science describes the existence of electromagnetic fields or force fields of energy around every object in the Universe. Each object vibrates at a different frequency and communicates with us via our senses.

This *Life Force Energy,* also referred to as Chi (Chinese), Ki (Japanese), or Prana (Indian), is transmitted through the body's energy centers.

There are seven primary energy centers, or chakras, that are natural force fields located over specific areas in the body. The word *chakra* comes from Sanskrit and refers to a spinning wheel. The chakras are conical in shape, with the point (vortex) of the cone being closest to the body; much like the point of a tornado is closest to the earth. The swirling vortex pulls energy into the body and releases energy from the body through the cone.

The chakras are the master coordinating centers for organizing the flow of physical, spiritual, and emotional energy, both the transmission from our bodies and the receiving into our life force. Think of the body as having a constantly changing series of seven energy fields that send and receive vibrations.

For centuries, Eastern cultures, most notably Traditional Chinese Medicine (TCM), have understood the concept of energy flow throughout the body and have documented the energy meridians and acupuncture points using techniques to increase body harmony, physical improvement, and emotional health.

The energy that runs through the chakras remains constant, although it increases or decreases with your actions, your thoughts, and whether your life is balanced and in harmony. Your emotions are projected out via the vibrations transmitted through the chakras and then resonate in your energy field. The energy that you receive back through the chakras triggers your emotional response.

Disharmony, emotional upset, or turbulent feelings all register in your force field. The expression, "I'm getting bad vibes about this" refers to a feeling or reaction, which is really a sensory input to the electromagnetic frequency of a person or situation within your own energy field.

A key to releasing emotional patterns and influencing spiritual awakening is the ability to change your vibes, which means altering your energy field or tuning in to new frequencies. So many times I have said to anyone who would listen, "It's in my energy field. What I am doing is what I am attracting. I know that, but I don't know how to change the energy that I give off so that I can change the energy that is coming my way."

That energy is what our emotions respond to. How do we make that shift? The energy we see, feel, hear, taste, touch and smell becomes our mirror.

Essential oils interact harmoniously with your energy field. The frequencies of the essential oils have the ability to transmute the discord, release the negative energy, and restore the chakra energies to balance. For instance, using the essential oil blend of **Harmony** on the energy centers helps to balance the body, enhance the healing process, and facilitate the release of stored emotions.

Locating the Chakras

Most of the focus on healing through the chakras is on the seven major points beginning at the base of the spine and ascending up the center line of the body to the crown. Chakras are numbered one through seven, identified by names, and closely associated with the colors of the rainbow.

Seven Major Chakras

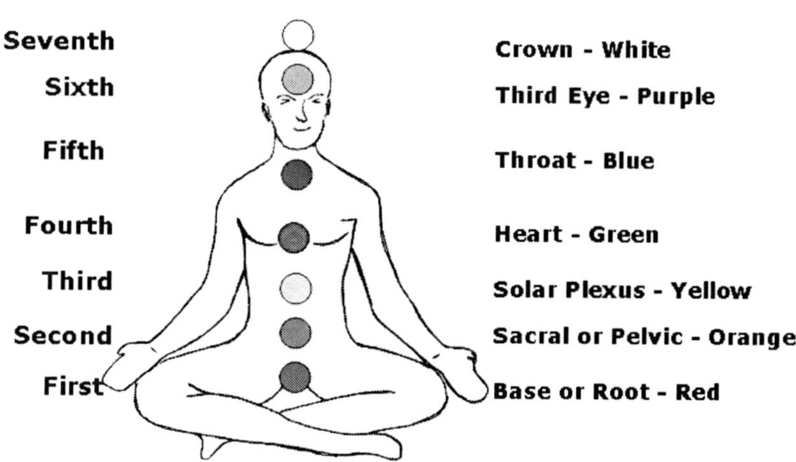

The first chakra, also called Base or Root, is at the base of the spine in the groin area at the tip of the coccyx, anatomically referred to as the pelvic floor. The second chakra, designated as Sacral or Pelvic, is located within the lower abdomen in the region of the female reproductive organs. The Solar Plexus or third chakra resonates in the upper abdomen just below the sternum (breastbone). The Heart or the fourth chakra lies in the area of the chest and heart. The area of the thyroid at the lower throat is designated as the fifth or Throat chakra. Situated in the middle of the forehead above the eyebrows is the Third Eye or sixth chakra. The seventh chakra or Crown resides at the top of the head.

Chakra Colors and Energy Fields

The spinning wheels of the chakras rotate with increasing speed from the Base to the Crown, with the Root chakra having the lowest frequency and the Crown chakra having the highest frequency.

The chakras are typically represented by the colors of the rainbow, with the shades advancing from red, orange, yellow, green, blue, purple, and then white at the Crown. The different wavelengths of the colors correspond to the frequency of the energy centers with the lower to higher vibrations.

The **Seven Major Chakras** diagram represents a simplified version of the way the chakra colors actually appear and is idealized to represent a healthy person. In fact, the force fields of spiraling energy extend well beyond the physical body. The energy of the chakras overlap, some fields being stronger than others, and this combined multitude of colors with the different wavelengths of light is known as your aura.

The aura is a personal electromagnetic profile, shaped like an eggshell, surrounding each of us and reflecting the subtle life energies within the body. Your aura changes moment to moment as your senses activate and your emotions trigger. Many Western and Eastern physicians have reported that they can feel as well as see these energy centers.

Everyone's aura is different, and everyone's aura changes instantaneously as we interact and evolve physiologically, spiritually, and emotionally.

Kirlian photography captures the picture of someone's aura at a particular point in time and is commonly used at metaphysical fairs. Originally developed by a Russian Technician in 1939, it employs a method to detect a high frequency charge and displays the colors through a Polaroid camera base.

Harmonic Convergence

The term, harmonics, is used to describe the effect of electrical loads converging on the same system from different sources and on different frequencies. In essence, harmonics are the conflicting frequencies of power.

In the case of the human body, the chakras are in a state of constant flux given the ebb and blow of the harmonics or life force energies. When harmonic convergence occurs, the resulting united force strengthens the energy field, balances the emotional energy, and supports the soul.

The chakras are your spiritual circuits connecting your physical body and your soul, with the energies constantly interacting. These energy centers act as conduits for the spiritual and emotional interactions to take place. Emotional energy is taken up by the body through the chakras and dispersed via energy channels called meridians.

Keeping them charged and in balance facilitates the energy flow and presents the opportunity for you to connect into your intuitive power, to feel, see, hear, and know. This will become clearer in the next chapter.

The lower chakras (one, two, and three) deal primarily with matter and form, the body, and connectedness to the material world. They are about physical, external, and human interaction. The upper chakras (five, six, and seven) are formless and act more in the etheric realms, the enlightened spirit. The higher frequencies of the upper energy centers correspond to elevated planes of spiritual existence. The heart, or fourth chakra, acts as the intermediary between the material and the etheric, the form and the formless. Think of the heart as the bridge between the upper and lower chakras.

The **Chakra Life Force Energy** diagram shows the connections between the first and seventh, second and sixth, and third and fifth chakras. While the fourth chakra is the heart of the matter, the forces of the other chakras create the harmonic convergence when aligned and balanced with the heart.

Chakra Life Force Energy

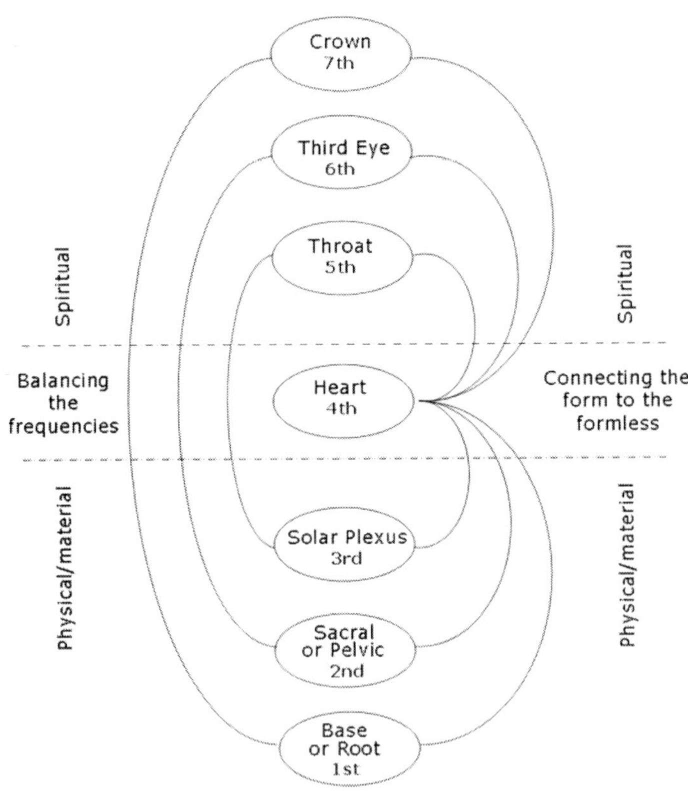

Corresponding and oppositional chakra frequencies for balance and harmonic convergence

Essential Oils for Harmonic Convergence

Using essential oils to balance and harmonize chakra energy combines the life force energy of the oils to act as catalysts to effect changes in your energy field. Adding essential oils to alternative healing methods heightens the experience for emotional freedom and spiritual evolvement.

In the descriptions below, there are a number of essential oils that may apply to different aspects of a specific chakra. Find the attribute or chakra that best fits your situation, select an essential oil or an oil blend from the list, and apply that oil to the designated chakra. At the end of the chakra descriptions is a section on *Chakra Balancing*; at the end of the chapter, look for *Putting It All Together.*

Essential oils and blends that benefit all of the chakras include **Awaken**, **Egyptian Gold**, **EndoFlex**, **Gratitude**, **Harmony**, **Inner Child**, **Peace & Calming**, **Present Time**, **Transformation**, **Valor**, **White Angelica**, **dorado azul**, and **lavender**.

First Chakra: Base or Root

This chakra relates to being anchored or grounded to the earth. It controls vitality, passion, belief patterns, self identity, and reflexes. Our sense of belonging to family and identifying with group characteristics is a key component. This is the form of energy that we feel when we are in a group that is rallied around the same cause, such as a sports event, a ceremony, or a riot. Mental and emotional stability are built (or dishonored) as we learn to communicate and perform within the family and group functioning.

Location – Pubic bone, base of coccyx

Color – Red represents a passion for life, stimulates energy and enthusiasm, releases fears and anxiety, and encourages action and confidence

Indications – Affects the sacrum, legs, feet, bones, rectum, and male sexual organs

Possible Physical Dysfunction - Rectal disorders, constipation, diarrhea, lower back pain, sciatica, varicose veins, prostrate problems, and male sexual disorders

Possible Mental-Emotional Issues - Paranoia, loss of will to live or being overly concerned with one's survival, reacting defensively to situations, feeling self-supported to stand up for self, ability to make day-to-day decisions, jungle mentality, and self-centeredness

Possible Life Lessons - Matters relating to the material world (being poor or being materialistic), individuality (knowing who you are), accepting and knowing that you have the right to success, well-being, groundedness, stability or security, courage, and patience

Oil Blends - Grounding, Valor, Di-Gize, ImmuPower, Acceptance, Gratitude, Gathering, Forgiveness, Peace & Calming, Transformation, Trauma Life, Release, Inner Child, SARA, and Mister

Single oils - cedarwood, lavender, cypress, patchouli, sandalwood, and vetiver

Second Chakra: Sacral or Pelvic

This powerful energy center is sometimes referred to as the Universal Life Force area, which supplies inner strength. It governs desires, emotions, sexuality and sexual magnetism, addictions, partnerships, and relationships. The physical power of this chakra takes on the forms of materialism, financial stability, physical survival, ownership, and authority.

Location - Pelvic area one to two inches below the navel, in the area of the ovaries or the bladder

Color - Orange represents warmth, evokes strong positive or negative responses, enhances visibility, and encourages social interaction

Indications - Affects the hip area, female reproductive organs, urinary tract and bladder, large intestine, appendix, immune system, lumbar vertebrae, and sensual emotions

Possible Physical Dysfunction **-** Colitis, irritable bowel syndrome, sexual dysfunction, chronic lower back issues, candida, bladder and urinary tract infections, intestinal mal-absorption, arthritis, and disorders related to the immune system

Possible Mental-Emotional Issues - Ethics and honor in or concerns with relationships, connections and friendships with others, the need to have power and control over the functioning of our physical environment (money, authority, and other people), blame and guilt, money and sex, overindulgence, confusion or loss of purpose, jealousy, envy, desire to possess, fear of losing control, out of proportion or cycling thoughts or reactions to external stimuli, hypochondria, feelings of isolation or wanting to be alone, fight or flight sensations, and overwhelming need to attract attention

Possible Life Lessons – Giving and receiving, acceptance of change, assimilation of new ideas, tolerance, surrender or forgiveness, working harmoniously and creatively with others, acceptance of self, acceptance of positive emotions such as love, pleasure, and desire

Oil Blends – Abundance, Acceptance, Believe, Clarity, Gentle Baby, Grounding, Forgiveness, Highest Potential, Joy, Juva Cleanse, Juva Flex, Live With Passion, Magnify Your Purpose, Purification, Trauma Life, Release, Sensation, and Surrender

Single Oils - bergamot, cistus, geranium, jasmine, melissa, myrrh, peppermint, rose, valerian, and ylang ylang

Third Chakra: Solar Plexus

This chakra is the energy center of personal power, ambition, and intellect, emotions based on intellect, external self-expression, personality, and ego. The self-assessment of emotions or inner beliefs are evaluated based on outside sources or surroundings and the recognition of the causal relationships between internal and external conflicts. The individual personal power (self-esteem, personality, and ego) views itself in relationship to the external world.

Location - Solar plexus area

Color - Yellow is mentally stimulating, encouraging creative thoughts and communication, inspiring a positive outlook, happiness, and enlightenment

Indications – The most common site for energy blocks; vitalizes major organs, including stomach, small intestine, liver, gall bladder, kidneys, spleen, adrenals, and pancreas

Possible Physical Dysfunction - Ulcers, adrenal overload, fatigue, general weakness or malaise, diabetes, pancreatitis, hepatitis, chronic or acute digestive problems, and liver dysfunction

Possible Mental-Emotional Issues – Challenged personal boundaries (trust, fear, and intimidation), insecure or overly concerned with self image (self-esteem, self-confidence, self-respect), feelings of inferiority or superiority, ineffective or domineering decision making, over controlling or lack of will power, submission to or domination over others, abuse of others, attempting to overachieve in an effort to be accepted, unfulfilled feelings of action, inability to achieve goals, not meeting responsibilities, fear of rejection, and sensitivity to criticism, authority, or ego expression by others

Possible Life Lessons – Acceptance of the human experience, conscious responsibility, self love, self control, soul understanding, humor, laughter, mastery of desire, letting go of ego, acceptance of self worth, ability to receive help from others, transformation, and hope

Oil Blends – Aroma Life, Australian Blue, Believe, Clarity, Di-Gize, Envision, En-R-Gee, Forgiveness, GLF, Highest Potential, Hope, Humility, ImmuPower, Into the Future, Joy, Juva Cleanse,

Juva Flex, Longevity, Magnify Your Purpose, Motivation, SARA, Release, Thieves, Transformation, and Trauma Life

Single Oils – Idaho balsam fir, cedarwood, chamomile (Roman), frankincense, palo santo, peppermint, melissa, sandalwood, spearmint, valerian, and vetiver

Fourth Chakra: Heart

The heart chakra sits in the middle of the others and acts to join together the body and the spirit. This point of connection with the Universal Life Force provides for opening within ourselves the space for conscious compassion, the integration of love, and spirituality.

Fourth chakra energy magnifies our emotional development. It is through the energy of this chakra that we become emotionally liberated by accepting that our personal and emotional challenges are part of the Universal or Divine plan. With the knowledge that this plan is intended to benefit our soul's conscious evolution, we can let go of the need to know why things have happened as they have. By accepting that this plan is pre-ordained, we can release the emotional pain and learn from our experiences, rather than blame our situation. An inner sense of harmony and peace surfaces when we embrace forgiveness, release judgment, and let go of the need for justice.

Through this amazing self-actualization, the heart chakra opens and gives out love and compassion. The upper and lower chakras open further and become more balanced as they are empowered from the heart.

Location - In the center of the chest at the level of the heart

Color - Green represents tranquility, healing, ease, and calm, with a sense of renewal and harmony

Indications - It is the area that vitalizes the heart, ribs, breasts, bronchia, lungs, diaphragm, shoulders, arms, hands, thoracic vertebrae, circulatory system, blood and cellular structures, and thymus

***Possible Physical Dysfunction* -** Physical heart ailments, bronchial pneumonia/bronchitis, lung cancer, asthma, breast cancer, circulatory problems, immune response disorders, rotator cuff (shoulder), arms, carpal tunnel (wrists), hands, and thoracic vertebrae

***Possible Mental-Emotional Issues* -** Ability to express or receive love, lack of self love or self-centeredness, emotional inner conflicts, attempting to control others or situations, anger or hatred, resentment, bitterness, self-judgment or judging others, feelings of disharmony, life-limiting or negative expressions, a limited focus of life, and feeling out of balance

Possible Life Lessons – Forgiveness, understanding, unconditional love, compassion, harmony, acceptance, peace, balance, contentment, and hope and trust

Oil Blends – Abundance, Acceptance, Australian Blue, Aroma Life, Awaken, Believe, Christmas Spirit, Clarity, Dream Catcher, Envision, Evergreen Essence, Grounding, Hope, Humility, Inner Child, Inspiration, Into the Future, Joy, Live With Passion, Magnify Your Purpose, Surrender, Sensation, 3 Wise Men, and Trauma life

Single Oils - bergamot, cedarwood, elemi, frankincense, geranium, helichrysum, jasmine, marjoram, palo santo, rosewood, sandalwood, and ylang ylang

Fifth Chakra: Throat

Located at the throat, the fifth chakra is naturally called the message center because it is the energetic point for transmitting verbal communications. Expression, including speech, art, singing, music, and creative writing, is manifested through the throat chakra.

The throat is also considered your willpower energy center. Your personal strength is measured by how well you exert control over yourself rather than how strong your need to exert your will over others. Under the Divine or Universal plan, you alone have the responsibility and accountability for yourself, your actions, feelings, and decisions. You are not intended to be controlled by others, just as they are not in charge of controlling you.

Through self-expression we learn the power of choice. This personal responsibility includes not blaming others for our emotional reactions to them or other external stimuli. We do not control the feelings and responses of others; rather, we are in charge of ourselves through willpower and self-choice. Understanding and managing our verbal responses is the strength of the fifth chakra.

Location - At the center of the neck, at the Adam's apple, above the collarbone

Color - Blue represents security, confidence, trustworthiness, accomplishment, calm, and knowledge, and is known to aid intuition

Indications - It is the area that vitalizes the throat and jaw areas, thyroid and parathyroid glands, hypothalamus, trachea, esophagus, cervical vertebrae, vocal cords, mouth, the breath, and the parasympathetic (involuntary) nervous system

Possible Physical Dysfunction – Thyroid problems, sore throat, laryngitis, swollen glands, mouth and gum disorders, temporomandibular joint issues, metabolic disorders, and immune system problems

Possible Mental-Emotional Issues – Issues around all verbal communication, difficulty or inability to express inner feelings, afraid to speak up, depression, lack of discernment, difficulty in communicating with clear expression, ineffective communications of thoughts and ideas, short periods of extreme emotion, being judgmental or critical, and feelings of worry, fear or paranoia

Possible Life Lessons – Conscious self control, allowing creative expression, integration of and living according to the truth, peace and knowledge, gentleness, kindness, honesty, reliability, loyalty, and understanding that the power of the spoken word is either a potential act of grace or a potential weapon

Oil Blends – Abundance, Acceptance, Australian Blue, Believe, Clarity, Dream Catcher, Envision, En-R-Gee, Exodus II, Gathering, Highest Potential, Hope, Humility, ImmuPower, Inspiration, Into the Future, Joy, Live With Passion, Longevity, Magnify Your Purpose, Melrose, Motivation, Purification, Raven, RC, RutaVaLa, SARA, 3 Wise Men, Thieves, and Trauma Life

Single oils - balsam fir, basil, cedarwood, cypress, eucalyptus blue, eucalyptus radiata, frankincense, marjoram, melaluca, oregano, peppermint, rosewood, sandalwood, spearmint, thyme, valerian, and vetiver

Sixth Chakra: Third Eye

This is the energy center of wisdom. The sixth chakra is the focal point for intuitive awareness, the connection to psychic power, inner vision, and spiritual insight. It is the nucleus for higher intuitive information (Higher Source) and opens to spiritual guidance in the form of thoughts, pictures, or wisdom. It also helps to release negative tendencies and selfish attitudes.

Location – From the front, it is located between the eyebrows and about one finger width above them. On the back of the body, the corresponding location is in the area of the medulla oblongata (the base of the brain stem)

Color - Purple represents wisdom and spirituality, and is calming to the mind and nerves, stimulating creativity

Indications – This area vitalizes the brain, eyes, ears, nose, sinuses, spinal cord, sympathetic nervous system (fight or flight), and the powerful pineal gland (which controls production of melatonin and coordinates fertility hormones)

Possible Physical Dysfunction - Symptoms of stress and tension, headaches, vision problems, sinusitis, major endocrine irregularity, lack of dreams or nightmares, neurological imbalances, ear or hearing disturbances, brain tumors, strokes, seizures, and learning disabilities

Possible Mental-Emotional Issues – Unwillingness or inability to see something that is important to your future advancement, feeling that you are at a dead end, overly detached or not grounded to the world, inability to concentrate, feeling that you have no intuition, lacking imagination to define your life goals, feeling you must intellectualize and control the outcome of your actions, blocked or overly active imagination, overly idealistic, and constant excessive expression of your ideas and thoughts

Possible Life Lessons – Opening to ideas from the wisdom of your inner self and from others, self-realization, self-esteem, feeling adequate, imagination, concentration, becoming a visionary, peace of mind, and the insight and ability to learn from experience

Oil Blends – Acceptance, Australian Blue, Awaken, Believe, Brain Power, Christmas Spirit, Citrus Fresh, Clarity, Dream Catcher, Envision, En-R-Gee, Evergreen Essence, Forgiveness, Gathering, Grounding, Highest Potential, Inspiration, Into the Future, Joy, Longevity, Magnify Your Purpose, Motivation, Surrender, RutaVaLa, Sacred Mountain, and 3 Wise Men

Single oils – Idaho balsam fir, bergamot, cedarwood, cypress, elemi, frankincense, geranium, helichrysum, melissa, mountain savory, peppermint, rose, rosewood, sandalwood, spearmint, and ylang ylang

Seventh Chakra: Crown

The seventh chakra is where the spirit and the mind integrate, nourishing and linking to the physical body. We are chakra connected to the higher dimensions of consciousness, internal awareness, spirituality, enlightenment, inspired thought, and higher frequencies—thus symbolizing the transcendental through prayer and meditation. The seventh chakra is typically open in people who are religious, or who have psychic or intuitive powers such as clairvoyance and claircognizance (see Chapter 5).

Location - At the crown or top of the head

Color – White helps with mental openness, encourages purity and clarity of thought, and helps to release clutter or obstacles in order to create new beginnings

Indications - Balancing the seventh chakra helps to integrate the right and left brain hemispheres; the energy influences the pituitary (the master endocrine gland)and hypothalamus gland (an important part of the limbic system or emotional brain), the musculoskeletal system, the skin, and the central nervous system

***Possible Physical Dysfunction* -** Cerebral disorders, mental exhaustion caused by non-physical symptoms, and intense reactions or sensitivities to light or sound

Possible Mental-Emotional Issues – Lack of inspiration, psychosis, confusion, alienation, self-defeated attitude, egotistical expressions such as vanity and pride or when false ideals become an intrinsic part of self, feelings of confusion, depression or uncertainty about things in life, inability to recognize truth around self-limiting concepts or materialistic consumption, confusion in recognizing reality, feeling of aloneness, need for power and control

Possible Life Lessons – Integration of Higher Source, connection with life and those around us, renewed identity, understanding, wisdom, faith, inner guidance, insight, and selfless service

Oil Blends – Acceptance, Australian Blue, Awaken, Brain Power, Christmas Spirit, Clarity, Dream Catcher, Envision, En-R-Gee, Evergreen Essence, Grounding, Highest Potential, Hope, Humility, Inspiration, Into the Future, Magnify Your Purpose, Sacred Mountain, and 3 Wise Men

Single oils – Idaho balsam fir, cedarwood, chamomile (Roman), frankincense, helichrysum, palo santo, melissa, myrrh, rose, rosewood, and sandalwood

Chakra Balancing

In order to achieve energy convergence (chakra balancing) it is best to work with all of the chakras at the same time. Otherwise, there is a risk of one or more chakras being out of balance with the others.

Essential oils and blends that benefit all of the chakras are **Awaken**, **Egyptian Gold**, **EndoFlex**, **Gratitude**, **Harmony**, **Inner Child**, **Peace & Calming**, **Present Time**, **Transformation**, **Valor**, **White Angelica**, **dorado azul**, and **lavender**.

Based on the **Chakra Life Force Energy** diagram and the chakra definitions, consider the following techniques for balancing chakras:

- Find the attribute or chakra that best fits your situation and choose the essential oils or oil blends from the list. Then identify the corresponding chakra and check if there is an oil blend or single oil from the list that resonates with you.

- Begin conscious breathing. Allow the flow of the Universe, your Higher Source, and the Guides or Angels that you might call on to assist you in this process. Let your breath be regular and steady, but remain conscious of it flowing in and out of your body. Feel it to the tips of your fingers and the ends of your toes.

- Apply the oils that you have chosen to the designated chakra, to the corresponding chakra, and to the heart.

- Balance the corresponding chakras with the energy from your hands. Use the right hand on the lower chakra and the left hand on the higher chakra. For example, place the fingers of your right hand on the third or Solar Plexus chakra and the fingers of your left hand on your throat or fifth chakra. Hold for about a minute or until you can feel the energetic connection.

- Now connect in to your heart energy. For chakras one through three, place your right hand on the lower chakra and your left hand on your heart. For chakras five through seven, place your right hand on your heart and your left hand on your chakra. The key to this hand placement is that your right hand is always lower or closer to your feet and your left hand is always higher or nearer to your head. Hold your hand positions until you can feel the energy balancing between the two points.

- Here is a technique that I use at the end of every massage. After applying the essential oil, I place my right fingers lightly on the heart chakra and my left index and forefingers on the crown chakra. This creates a sense of harmony, uniting the brain and the heart.

- When you feel that you are complete with the experience, begin conscious breathing. Lightly cup your hands over your nose and mouth so that you have the opportunity to inhale the oils that are on your hands. This is the way to get the most benefit. Slowly come back to reality.

The Physiological Connection

Physiologically, each of the seven chakras is located at the relative anatomical position of an endocrine gland (the glands that regulate the physical and emotional processes in the body) and represents the swirling energy of the effects of the hormone released by that gland. These hormone-producing glands of the endocrine system are the gonads (testes and ovaries), pancreas, adrenals, thymus, thyroid, parathyroid, pineal, hypothalamus, and pituitary.

The pituitary is often called the master gland and, working in concert with the hypothalamus, exerts a wide range of control over the endocrine system.

The limbic area (see Chapter 2) is the hormone-producing system of the brain. It includes the amygdala, hippocampus, pineal, pituitary, thalamus, and hypothalamus. Essential oils increase circulation of oxygen to the brain. This better enables the pituitary and other glands to secrete neural transmitters and hormones that support the endocrine and immune systems.

The thyroid is one of the most important glands for regulating body systems. The hypothalamus plays an even more important role since it regulates the thyroid, adrenals, and pituitary.

Chakras and Endocrine Glands

	Chakra	**Location**	**Gland**
Seventh	Crown	Top of head	Pituitary Hypothalamus
Sixth	Third Eye	Forehead	Pineal
Fifth	Throat	Throat	Thyroid Parathyroid
Fourth	Heart	Chest	Thymus
Third	Solar plexus	Upper abdomen	Adrenals Pancreas
Second	Sacral or Pelvic	Pelvis	Ovaries
First	Base	Groin	Testes

These endocrine glands regulate the electrical frequency throughout the physical body. When the body is out of balance, much of the cause of that imbalance is in the endocrine system. Starting a chakra harmonizing session with the **EndoFlex** essential oil blend is a beautiful way to signal to the body that the balancing act is about to begin.

Auricular Chakra Technique

Chakras may also be balanced by using the acupressure or auricular points on the ear. Auriculotherapy, which was developed in France during the mid 20th century, is a modality wherein points on the external surface of the ear, or auricle, are activated to relieve conditions in other areas of the body. There are over 2,700 points of stimulation on the ear.

This is a similar concept to reflexology, which uses acupressure points on the hands and the feet, but is eminently more complex. Auriculotherapy practitioners stimulate the auricular points with acupuncture needles, acupressure, or electrical frequency.

Auriculotherapists believe that the ears are the "keyboard and monitor to the brain"—an interesting concept when you think of stimulating auricular points with essential oils. In auriculotherapy, the left ear is considered the emotional ear and the right ear is designated as the physical ear. I have found it most effective to open and balance the relevant chakras applying essential oils to the ear reference points.

Auricular Chakras

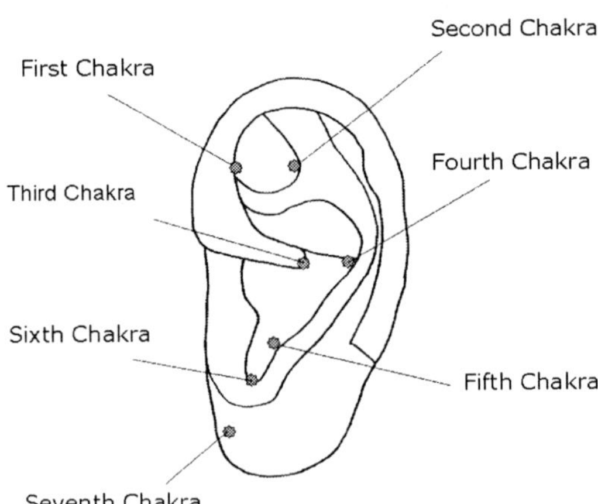

The chakras are represented on each ear as indicated in the **Auricular Chakra** chart[1] above.

1 With permission from Elsevier Limited

Locate the Chakras that Need Balancing

We can use the auricular points to determine the chakras that need balancing.

- Use a blunt object such as a wooden matchstick, the eraser-end of a pencil, or the handle of a toothbrush to palpate the auricular chakra points.

- Test both ears. With gentle but firm pressure on each point, notice any tenderness. That sensitivity is an indication of chakra imbalance—if it hurts, it is out of balance. Use that information to balance the chakras as indicated with the previous *Chakra Balancing* method or follow the technique below.

With the knowledge that the left ear represents emotion and the right ear is designated as the physical, make note of the chakra points, for each ear, that appear out of balance. Look back over the chakra descriptions for clues and insights as to what may be blocking your emotional or physical energy.

Balance the Chakras Using Auricular Points

We can balance the chakras using the auricular points, either using the ears alone or in synchronicity with the actual chakra locations. Balance both ears.

- Place a drop of the chosen oil in your non-dominant hand and rub clockwise three times with the forefinger of your other hand to energize the oil.

- Place your forefinger with the oil on it at the location of the auricular chakra point. Put your thumb behind your ear if needed for stabilization. With firm and steady pressure, hold for 30 seconds. Do not press so hard that your ear hurts.

Putting it all Together

Balancing or creating harmony in the chakras is not as difficult as some energy practitioners would have you believe. Energy workers love to talk about your energy centers being out of balance as though it is a great mystery.

At any given point in time, you will have one or more chakras in control or dominate. That is normal—it goes with the ebb and flow of who you are.

Just as you might have a weak link in your anatomy—as in "Every time I get overly tired or stressed, my eye twitches," you also will have weak links in your chakra system. After studying the chakras, you might discover that you are pre-disposed to a certain stumbling block or a pre-determined emotional reaction when a certain chakra is out of balance.

Use this information for identifying your areas of life enhancement. If you know, for instance, that some of your central issues are in the area of the fifth chakra, and you have the information that the corresponding third chakra creates harmonic convergence when balanced with the heart, you now have empowerment to change your circumstances.

Honor you intuition for your energy balancing.

Chapter 5

Your Soul's Consciousness

Soul Wisdom

We have all heard stories of someone who is a gifted healer, a remarkable intuitive, or who has psychic powers.

Some people come into this world with amazing talents in the psychic or intuitive realms, just as others are born with different astonishing gifts. For example, my sister-in-law's mother could hear a song once and then play it on the piano perfectly. Think of opera singers, dancers, or athletes. A friend of mine has a photographic memory.

What sets them apart from the rest of us? Nothing!

We all have intuitive or psychic abilities from birth—we are born ready. But for most of us, our current culture requires that we fit into patterns or norms that do not encourage the use of these faculties. The skills simply become dormant from lack of use.

We just need a little help in understanding how intuitive feelings work, and then we need the patience and the appreciation to recognize that capacity in ourselves. Just like any other skill, we improve with practice.

Being intuitive means connecting into and listening to your soul's wisdom—your Higher Source. Learning to trust in your Higher Source has many benefits, including feeling better about yourself, having more confidence with improved self-esteem, having better decision making skills with greater understanding of circumstances and events, having increased awareness, grounding, and control, having less fear of situations, and maintaining overall peace and balance.

Trust Your Intuition

The previous chapter on chakras discussed the concept of the human energy field. This energy field is alive and contains information as it pulsates or vibrates with varying frequencies based on the body's physiological or biological processes. Your energy field extends out as far as your outstretched arms, running the full length of your body and transmits messages and receives signals through your senses.

This sending and receiving of electricity to and from other people's bodies becomes the constant information exchange with everything around us, and this is what intuitives perceive.

Intuition is the knack of picking up or distinguishing Life Force Energy. You can probably use your intuitive sense to a certain degree—we all do—but you can learn to tap into your innate capacity, your Higher Source, more quickly and at any time.

We all receive information in different ways, depending on our specific psychic strength and our connection to our senses. It is the right brain that governs intuition and enhances the ability to tune into psychic ability.

There are six recognized techniques or senses. The senses are special intuitive methods for gaining information. Most people draw on more than one sense in using their intuitive abilities. Practice helps develop these talents and to identify with more than one.

Clairvoyance comes from the French meaning *clear seeing* and is the capacity to focus on or gain information through means other than from the normal five human senses. This is sometimes called second sight or spiritual communication. Prophets are considered to be clairvoyant, but everyone possesses this talent on some level. For instance, from 9/11, there are many personal stories that tell of individuals changing their plans at the last minute, thus averting certain death.

Clairsentience is sometimes referred to as extra-sensory perception (ESP). It happens when a person feels knowledge or information through the vibrational energy of other people. Clairsentient individuals might sense something physical. For example, medical intuitives have the ability to tune into malfunctioning organs or systems in another person's body. Empathic individuals, also known as empaths, pick up on the thoughts and emotions of others.

Clairaudience is the ability to acquire information by auditory means. Generally these people are the only ones who can hear or perceive sounds such as voices, noises, or other subtle tones. A clairaudient person might even hear the voices or thoughts of spirits of persons who are deceased.

Clairalience happens when a person acquires psychic knowledge primarily by means of smelling. Because of smell's strong association with emotions (please see Chapter 2), aromatherapy increases our intuitive abilities on all levels. People who use unadulterated essential oils over a period of time hone this skill, and it feeds or opens the other senses.

Clairgustance is an intuition in which a person may taste a substance without putting anything in their mouth. Those who have this ability claim that through taste, they are able to perceive the essence of a substance from the spiritual or ethereal realms.

Claircognizance is a precognition by which a person acquires psychic or intuitive information by means of intrinsic knowledge. It is the ability to know something without knowing how or why you know it, sometimes referred to as "I just know." The adage, Think—Stop Thinking—Feel, is a way to describe how to enter this state of consciousness.

The concept of using essential oils to stimulate the opening or re-awakening of this innate intuitive ability that we all have cannot be underestimated. Chapter 3 discussed the frequency of essential oils and Chapter 4 listed essential oils for opening and clearing chakras. By raising the bodily frequency and focusing on clearing our energy fields, we have the ability to release from the subconscious those ideas, thoughts, dreams, and aspirations that we desire and to bring them into conscious alignment. This is not suggesting that the use of essential oils is the only means by which we can do this; rather, the oils are a beneficial tool in the quest for spiritual insight.

Tuning into Your Intuitive Sources

How do you get started? You might have read the above list and just knew that you were claircognizant. Congratulations! Here is an exercise that may assist you in gaining more insight into your personal path that will allow you to connect to your Higher Source and help you listen to your soul's wisdom.

Preparation

Listening is the key to tapping into your intuition. Be quiet and stop the mind chatter so that you can distinguish the messages coming from your Higher Source.

Find a comfortable place, a room that feels good, where you will not be disturbed. This place should feel safe and beckoning. Be sure that all phones are turned off so as to eliminate all outside distractions. Background music is not recommended, but is optional so long as it is quiet and helps you to get centered. It should be soothing to the soul. You will be doing a writing exercise, so have pen and paper handy, and be sure that you will be comfortable in this position for 15 to 20 minutes.

The essential oils that you will want to have close at hand are:

Oil Blends - Envision, Gratitude, 3 Wise Men, Valor, and White Angelica. Optional: Awaken, Believe, Grounding, Highest Potential, Inspiration, Magnify Your Purpose, Sacred Mountain, and Tranquil

Single Oils - dorado azul. Optional: cedarwood, Roman chamomile, and palo santo

- Start by applying **Valor** on the bottoms of both feet.

- Sit on the floor with your knees bent and the bottoms of your feet facing each other. Place three to six drops of **Valor** in your left hand. Using the fingertips of your right hand, stir the oil clockwise three times to energize the oil. Apply the oil to the bottom of your right foot. Do the same with the left foot. Now, hold the palms of your hands on the bottom of your feet with your right hand on your right foot and your left hand on your left foot. The palm of your hand should fit snugly at the arch of your foot, allowing your fingertips to curl around the outside of your feet. After a few minutes, you will feel the energy beginning to pulsate between your hands and your feet, especially in the area of your arches. Once you sense the balance in both hands, you are ready to move to the next step.

- Use **White Angelica** as your energy shield on your shoulders. This provides protection for your energy field as you tune into your Higher Source.

Place one to two drops of **White Angelica** in the palm of your left hand. Using the fingertips of your right hand, stir the oil clockwise three times to energize the oil. Using your fingers, apply the oil to the top of each shoulder, starting with the left shoulder. Then apply the oil to the middle of the sternum (breastbone) and finally to the entire length of the back of the neck.

- Place the essential oil blend of **3 Wise Men** on your crown and ear lobes, at the *Seventh Chakra Auricular Point*. Squeeze firmly with your thumb and forefinger and hold for 30 seconds.

Auricular Chakras

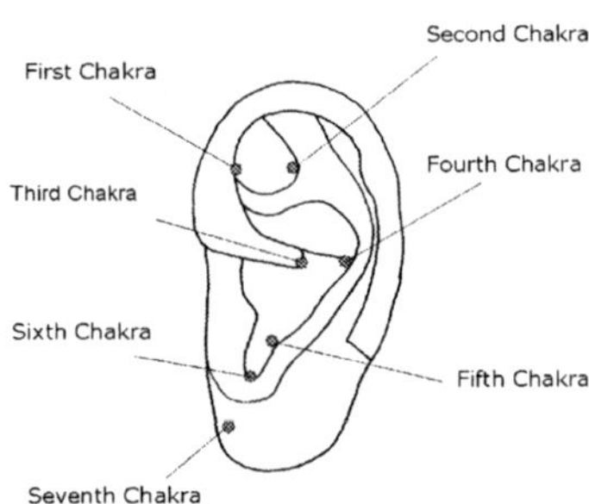

- Place the **Envision** or **Inspiration** essential oil blend on the *Sixth Chakra Auricular Point*. Again squeeze and hold for 30 seconds. Optionally place a drop on your Third Eye.

- Place a drop of **dorado azul** or **Believe** on the indentation at the base of the skull.

- Now, place a drop of **Gratitude** over your heart and rub clockwise three times.

- Sit quietly for a few minutes and breathe deeply with your eyes closed. Feel the breath encircling your body. Feel it reach your toes, the tips of your fingers, and the top of your head, all over. Check in with yourself to know that you feel safe and comfortable. If you need further assistance to get centered and focused, use some of the other oils mentioned above.

- With pen and paper (preferably not your keyboard) write a story. This could be a personal experience, an event that someone else had that moved you, or a fictional tale. Maybe you wish to write about your day, your recent vacation, or your most exhilarating experience. Take your time and spend at least 10 minutes doing this writing exercise.

- Write about what happened, your reaction to it, or what you encountered. Were you outside or inside? What was the weather like? Was it pastoral and serene or busy and hectic? Be as accurate and descriptive as possible. Don't try to make sense of the writing or worry about sentence structure or the flow of the story. It is important that you write continuously.

- If you get stuck, try putting the essential oil blend of **3 Wise Men** or **Sacred Mountain** on your Crown chakra. You might try **palo santo** right between your eyes at your Third Eye or the **Grounding** essential oil blend on the *Bubbling Spring* point on your feet.

Bubbling Spring

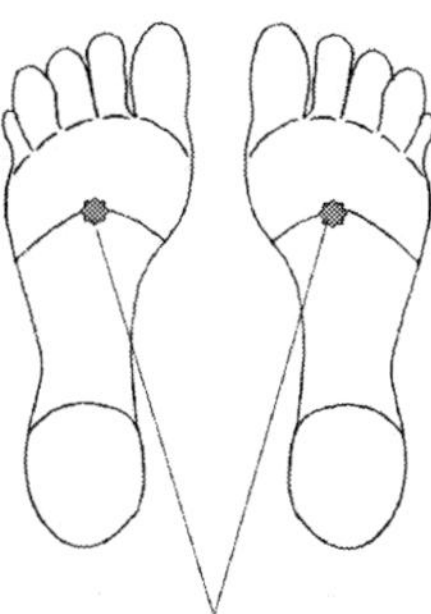

Bubbling Spring is a Chinese acupuncture point, *Kidney 1 (K 1).* It is located at the lowest energetic point in the body, on the bottom of the foot, behind the ball of the foot, in the depression in the center of the sole. It is our connection with the earth.

After applying the essential oil to K1, place your thumb on the point and alternately press and release in a pumping motion for 30 seconds to 1 minute. Repeat this press and release pumping motion on the other foot.

Complete this exercise before you read further. The explanation below may alter the way you write your story!

Interpreting Your Results

Now this is the fun part! Here comes the "Aha!" moment.

We all speak and write with terminology that facilitates our personal means of communicating by using the words that relate to our dominant precognition or intuitive powers.

How did you describe things in your story? Look at what you have written to find the sense (or senses) that appear the strongest.

For most of us, our most dominant sense is seeing, and we prefer visually descriptive words like, "I saw the tree in the meadow with the leaves rippling in the wind," or "When Beth came on the scene, everyone was hustling to get things ready."

The second most frequently interpreted sense is hearing. For example, "When I heard the thunder, I thought the dogs would howl," or "After all that walking yesterday, my knees were really barking at me."

Maybe you wrote, "When I heard the thunder, *I just knew* that the lightning would strike that tree."

We have been taught to express our feelings and emotions using phrases like, "I had a feeling that Marie and Liz would show up for dinner," or "A feeling of euphoria came over me when I won the lotto."

Some of us communicate in a more literal or sequential fashion. For instance, "After Susan washed the car, she went to the grocery store and then to the bank," or "When Theresa called me, I was in the middle of cleaning the kitchen."

Did your sense of touch tell you something about your situation or your surroundings? For example, "That was the best massage I ever had because your quality of touch is wonderful," or "When I caressed that flower, the softness of the petals was wondrous."

How about taste? "When I tasted the pie made with therapeutic grade essential oils, I was impressed at the depth and the quality of the flavors," or "The food that Jack prepared was sumptuous, and I did not want to stop eating."

Now take a moment to go back over your story and with a different colored pen, circle the words using the following as categories: seeing, feeling, touching, hearing, smelling, and tasting. Also use IJK for "I just know."

This is your opportunity to understand your foremost means of intuition. You will likely find that one category is used more frequently, but your other senses will be represented as well. This most often repeated sense is the one that you will practice listening and paying attention to because it facilitates your spiritual connection. In some cases, you may find that all of the categories are equally prevalent, which means that you are most likely Claircognizant.

Connecting to Your Higher Senses

Once you have mastered listening to the special sense of your Higher Source, you must then learn to trust what you hear. This is actually the harder of the two steps, as we are not familiar with trusting that which is intangible. The following descriptions and associated essential oils are intended to facilitate the process of listening and trusting.

Clairvoyance: Visualizing or Seeing

Very visual words or words that have a descriptive emphasis, portraying what you saw in the scene, indicate clairvoyance. Clairvoyants relate to images and symbols and are able to see things in their mind's eye. For example, they may be able to see a vision of an accident as it is happening in another location. Clairvoyants may have the ability to see another person's aura.

Essential oils to enhance clairvoyance are:

Oil Blends - 3 Wise Men, Sacred Mountain, and Believe

Single oils - sandalwood, **frankincense**, and **dorado azul**

Clairsentience: Feeling or Sensing

Feeling or seeing someone's aura or energy field is the specialty of the clairsentient. Feelings words mean that you are empathic. The expression, "I just had a feeling" is the hallmark of this precognition pattern. Clairsentients speak in touchy–feely terms and are usually found in the healing professions. They are emotionally gifted and remarkably intuitive healers (both allopathic and alternative). They sometimes become too connected with their patients.

The simple question, "How do you feel?" is an empathic one. However, a clairsentient will know the answer to the question even if you do not respond; they feel what is happening. Empaths pick up vibrations from objects by holding something in their hands, which is why clairsentients like to make physical contact to strengthen their connection.

Essential oils to enhance clairsentience are:

Oil Blends - Transformation, Harmony, Inner Child, Awaken, Gratitude, and Magnify Your Purpose

Clairaudience: Hearing

If your words relate to how things sound to you or what you heard, you are clairaudient. Music, chanting, and drumming are very useful tools to help strengthen the clairaudient's connection to their innate abilities. Many clairaudients gain great insight simply by listening to a person's voice. Their clues may also come from the loudest noises or a quiet and serene stillness.

Essential oils to enhance clairaudience include:

Oil Blends - Humility, Inspiration, Present Time, and **Thieves**

Clairalience: Smelling

Clairalient intuitives have a heightened sense of smell. Independent of the other senses, the sense of smell connects into the emotional portion of the brain. The limbic brain responds only to smell, not words—either spoken or written. Smell triggers the amygdala gland, which manages the storage and retrieval for all of your emotional experiences. Smell is capable of evoking memories and emotions of incidences that happened many years ago. For example, a memory triggered by a smell may be applicable to a present day situation in which you are required to take action.

Essential oils to enhance clairalience include:

Oil Blends - White Angelica, Juva Cleanse, Highest Potential, GLF, Sacred Mountain, and Aroma Life

Single oils - lemon, bergamot, and vitex

Clairgustance: Tasting

The Clairgustant is at home in the world of gastronomy. Perhaps subtler than others in terms of knowing, information comes to the intuitive through recognition or memory of a taste sensation. As with clairalience, aromatherapy can be especially useful for persons with clairgustance.

Essential oils to enhance clairgustance include:

Oil Blends - Valor, RutaVala, Humility, Egyptian Gold, Believe, Inner Child, and Exodus II

Claircognizance: Simply Knowing

Claircognizance is the intuitive gift of simply knowing without understanding how you know. Without relying on words, events, actions, things, or visualizing, you just know. The information is just there. In this form of precognition, the intuitive remains fully conscious (not in a trance). Learning to listen to and trust this sense is usually difficult, but once mastered, it is remarkable. Claircognizant individuals also tap into the other senses, meaning that there is a very intimate and close connection to their Higher Source.

Essential oils to enhance claircognizance include:

Oil Blends - Believe, Inner Child, Juva Cleanse, Egyptian Gold, Humility, and Sacred Mountain

Single Oils - dorado azul, palo santo, and bergamot

No one is limited to just one of these abilities, but one of your six senses will come more naturally to you than the others. Once you have determined which of the senses that you gravitate toward, you have a starting point for developing your communicating language and building your intuition. As you heighten your awareness, you will find yourself picking up on clues and messages from all of your senses. Learn to trust your intuition. It is a natural part of who you are.

To receive guidance for yourself, use your intuition by connecting to your Higher Source. It is this link and communication with your Higher Consciousness that is the distinction between psychic ability and the interconnectedness to your soul.

Verbal Fluency

Another gift of understanding the various senses is knowing that the inherent dominant intuition you use for connecting to your Higher Source is the same prevailing sense that you use for everyday verbal interactions. If you want to improve communications with others in the interest of developing closer or more personal relationships, listen carefully (even though you might not be clairaudient) to the words that the other person uses. Develop an awareness of another's preferred communication style. As you begin to relate to that person in their dominate sense, they will feel a much stronger bond with you because they will feel that you really understand them!

As an example, suppose that your significant other is looking for a new job. You might say (clairvoyant), "Clearly there are plenty of opportunities for you out there. You just have to look!" or (clairsentient), "I know that you can get this job. I sense it happening." In return they (clairaudient) might reply angrily or dejectedly, "You just don't listen to what I am telling you. I pounded the streets all day and got nothing!"

How many times have you had someone say to you, "You are not listening to me," or "You just don't listen"? That is because you are not speaking to them in the language that reflects their preferred sense or affirming their speech patterns. We want to be spoken to in the same language that we speak, in our preferred verbal skill set.

So if someone complains that we are not listening, that simply means one of two things. The first possibility is that we may really not be listening because we have a multitude of mind chatter (our own agenda) going on that prevents us from actually hearing and understanding them. The second possibility is that we may not be getting our message across to them because we are using a different language of communication than they are.

The identification of daily verbal interaction can be taken a step further. How does my verbal fluency interact with someone else's verbal platform? Can I adjust my verbal skills to communicate more freely, adroitly, fluently, interestingly, or educatedly with others so that they will continue a discourse that most interests me, them, us?

Relying on our self-wisdom, our link to our Higher Source, and understanding that these skills translate into normal daily dialogue goes a long way with regard to improving interpersonal relationships. But it also helps on a more intrinsic, subliminal, and subconscious level. Once we know our basic platform for communicating and are able to identify another person's pattern, we will feel the language differences between us. There is the freedom, the opportunity for growth, and the choice to make changes in our lives that we have not been able to make before.

Trust that you have this creative, intuitive ability and then listen to your Higher Source. Our precognitive power is sending us messages all of the time. Pay attention to the clues and acknowledge the wisdom. Heed the information that is coming to you from your soul. Be open, be aware, listen and trust.

Part 2

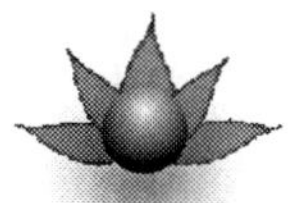

AromaMethods

Essential Oil Techniques

My experience in using therapeutic grade essential oils with any alternative methodology produces an outcome that is greatly enhanced. Essential oils facilitate the process, soothe the psyche, nurture the body, augment the energetic alignments, nurture the soul, and magnify whatever benefits are possible.

I hope that the techniques included here will encourage you to develop your own ideas for using essential oils. The techniques intentionally repeat the entire process for applying some of the oils and the illustrations also duplicate, so that you do not have to stop and look something up in the appendix.

The spiritual and emotional essential oil blends have names like **Joy, Harmony, Gratitude, Release**, and **Forgiveness**—names that mean something. But I always wondered how they could be put to practical everyday use to effect change, and I was determined to find out. This section of the book includes exercises that I have used as I experimented on myself. Most of the methods I have developed, while a few were developed by others.

I began by using **Inspiration**. That led me to an initial system of setting up all of the emotional and spiritual oils on a shelf where I could see them every day. Some days, I used just a single oil blend to see what effect it would have for the day. Other times I used a combination of oils. My method of selecting the oils was sometimes random, sometimes very specific, and sometimes intuitive.

Then I developed a systematic approach. Dowsing with a pendulum helped me to determine the oils that would maintain my highest good based on the intention that I set for the day. In addition to a pendulum, you can also approach many of these exercises using muscle testing. For more information on muscle testing or how to dowse with a pendulum, visit the website: www.aromatherapyforthesoul.com.

Consistency and repetition are necessary keys to success. Consider making a plan for the next three months and sticking to your intention no matter what. Keep a diary. Record how you feel at the beginning of your journey; include your current feelings about yourself and present situations. Describe your physical symptoms and rate the pain level on a scale from one to ten. As you try these exercises, keep frequent notes—daily or weekly—in your journal. Be sure to note your progress as it relates to your feelings, physical changes, and mental states. Keep track of the techniques and the oils that you use, and how you feel about the experience.

Remain objective and do not get discouraged. Avoid judging and comparing yourself from one day to the next. We all have ups and downs. If you have a day where you are disheartened, allow yourself to accept that feeling as a part of the human experience and appreciate that emotion for what it is. Do not dwell on it as a personal failure.

Instead, consider the following affirmation as a positive belief in yourself. Use the **Believe** essential oil blend on the back of your neck and say out loud, "I recognize and accept my lapse as a positive belief in my personal evolvement and my ability to move forward to the next excellent step." Relax and breathe into the moment after you say this.

Each of us, individually, is a powerful person on the planet. We dictate and describe our wholesomeness and our beingness as it relates to us. No one else has that responsibility or cares about us the way we care about ourselves.

How to Use the Oils

For all of the methods described below, use the essential oils as follows:

- Place a drop or two of oil in the palm of your left hand.
- Using the fingertips of your right hand, stir the oil clockwise three times to energize the oil.
- Apply the oil as indicated. In some cases, the technique may call for more than one or two drops of oil.

Method 1

Meditation

If you choose to meditate, there is no better companion than essential oils. I have included a sample meditation here and then a series of optional techniques to include as you customize your personal meditative experience.

Meditation assists in honing your intuitive skills when you tune into your Higher Source on a regular basis. It will help you to access your higher senses and provide the knowledge and understanding to open and balance your chakras.

Notes

Preparation

It is very important to choose your oils before you start, so that you are not interrupted during your quiet time. If you think that you may want alternative oils, have them ready also. If you are planning a contemplative experience around one of the six higher senses skills or one of the seven chakras, select multiple oils from the corresponding lists so that you have the options available to you at the time you want them.

Set your personal stage by finding quiet, peaceful, and comfortable surroundings, and know that you feel secure and relaxed in this space. Plan your session for the same time every day. Turn off all phones, pagers, and interruptive devices. You may wish to view lighted candles to add a point of focus or atmosphere. Soft, centering music in the background is optional, but not recommended because the essential oils you will be applying have vibrational energy.

When You Are Ready

- Begin by breathing easily.
- Apply **Valor** on the bottoms of both feet.

  Sit on the floor with your knees bent and the bottoms of your feet facing each other. Place three to six drops of **Valor** in your left hand. Using the fingertips of your right hand, stir the oil clockwise three times to energize the oil. Apply the oil to the bottom of your right foot, and then repeat the process for the left foot. Now, hold the palms of your hands on the bottom of your feet with your right hand on your right foot and your left hand on your left foot. The palm of your hand should fit snugly at the arch of your foot, allowing your fingertips to curl around the outside of your feet. After a few minutes, you will feel the energy beginning to pulsate between your hands and your feet, especially in the area of your arches. Once you sense the balance in both hands, you are ready to move to the next step.

Notes

- Use **White Angelica** to safeguard your energy field as you tune into your Higher Source.

  Using your fingers, apply the oil to the top of each shoulder, starting with the left shoulder. Then apply the oil to the middle of the sternum (breastbone) and finally to the entire length of the back of the neck.

- (Optional) Apply either **Australian Blue** or **Grounding** to the *Bubbling Spring Point* on the bottoms of the feet.

Bubbling Spring

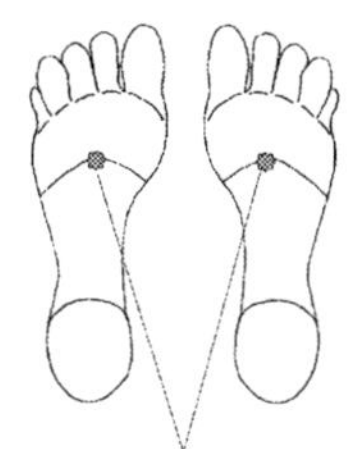

- Place the essential oil blend of **3 Wise Men** on your crown. Optionally, place the oil on the location of the seventh chakra on your ear lobes, squeezing firmly with your thumb and forefinger. Hold for 30 seconds.

Auricular Chakras

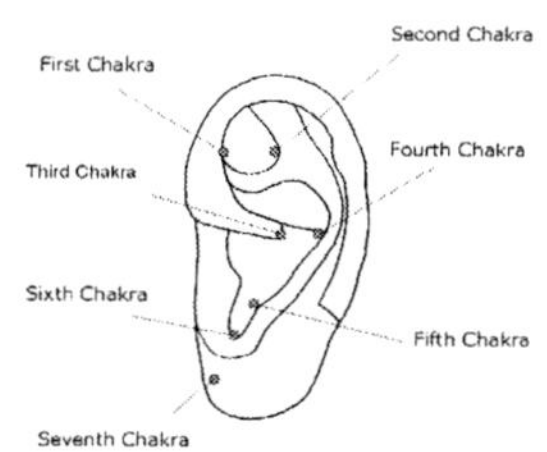

Notes

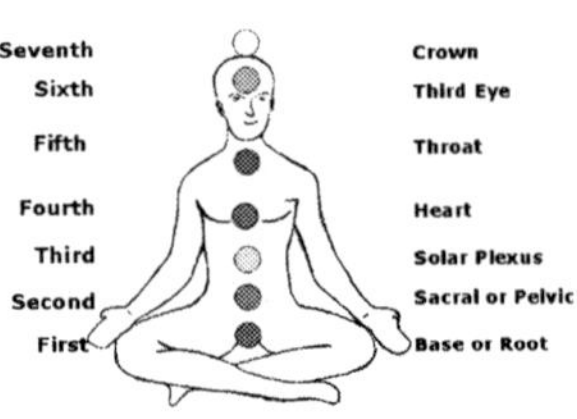

- Apply **Harmony** to the chakras, starting with the first and working in order to the seventh. You may wish to apply **Harmony** to the auricular chakra points also.
- Apply a drop of **dorado azul** or **Believe** in the indentation at the base of the skull.
- Place a drop of **Gratitude** over your heart and rub clockwise three times.
- Slowly count backwards from ten as you become centered and feel the emotional strength of the oils surrounding you with the peace and quietude. You may wish to close your eyes while doing this.
- Begin conscious breathing. Allow the flow of the Universe, your Higher Source, and the Guides or Angels that you might call on to assist you in this process. Let your breath be regular and steady, but remain conscious of it flowing in and out of your body. Feel it to the tips of your fingers and the ends of your toes.

When I meditate, I have a series of special Guides and Angels that I ask to be present to assist me. These amazingly beautiful and knowing spirits are with me all of the time and I know that they just need to be called upon to help me. (For instance, I just know that the Archangel Michael is one of my Guardian Angels.) On a subliminal level, I know their presence and respect that they are here to help me for my highest good. When I meditate and want to tune into my Spiritual Guides, I used to think about all of the different presences that I felt and perhaps even call them by name. That took time, so now I

Notes

use a shortcut. This might sound silly and even disrespectful, but it is meant with the best of intentions and it is quite effective. I simply say, "Hi Gang, I'm here, please let me know your presence." And I do know that they are tuned in because I generally get chills up and down my spine.

When I give a massage, I always call in my Higher Source, my Guides, and my *Healing Spirits.* These Healing Spirits are a special group of Master Healers that take over for me during the massage session and direct my intuition toward giving the most beneficial treatment for the person on the table.

When I am complete with my meditation or when the massage is over, I always thank my special Guides and Spirits for their help and guidance.

- Permit your thoughts to go to your favorite space, somewhere safe and comforting for you. Is it a sea shore, a quiet campsite in the mountains, the solitude of a lonely forest glade, or a beautiful flower garden? Seek peace and solitude. No one can harm you here.
- See shapes and colors, feel the breezes, and smell the air. Is the image floral, pastoral, or mountianeous? Do you smell the trees, sea breezes, or other fragrances?
- Feel and sense your breath. This is very important in meditation. Let your breathing lead you through your imaginary travels.

Notes

Customizing Your Meditation

At this point, begin the customization of your meditation experience. Select oils from the respective lists from Chapters 4 or 5 and proceed as follows:

The placement of the oils is your choice. Think about the chakra locations on the body and on the ears. Other options include your wrists, back of neck, temples, or the bottoms of your feet. You might focus your attention on your crown to activate your higher senses.

Allow your Spirit Guides to encourage you in the placement of the oils. This is an incredible opportunity to learn to trust in the oils and to trust in your spirit. Go with the flow, and allow the process to happen. During this time, your breathing should be slow and rhythmic.

❍ Affirmations

This would be a good time for expressing some pre-determined affirmations. Here are some ideas.

- I feel more relaxed.
- I am comfortable in my own body.
- I am at peace with my ___________ situation.
- I am my existence.
- I am the most important person in my life.

- I leave psychological self-absorption in order to attain spiritual self-awareness.
- I am feeling more peaceful.
- I am love, and I send love to all others in the Universe to whom I am connected.

❍ If you are looking for clarity around a situation or an issue, now would be an appropriate time to explore this. You may wish to apply the **Clarity** oil blend to your Third Eye and your ears. Listen for your answers. This is when you will receive hints or even direct messages. There may be flashes of insight or gut feelings. The answer that you are seeking may seem clouded in a puzzle or a fuzzy image. Stay focused and do not dismiss any or all silly thoughts. Ask,"What do I need to know?"

Your answer might not come right away. Have the **Surrender** oil blend handy. Apply it to whatever area on your body feels appropriate, and allow a few minutes of conscious breathing. If the answers are still not forthcoming, let go and continue with the wrap-up of your meditation. You might not be ready for the complete answers to your situation at this time. However, use the **Dream Catcher** oil blend before going to bed and pay close attention to your dreams for the next few nights or to your thoughts on the following mornings. Keep a pad and pen close at your bedside. The answer is closer than you think, just under the surface, waiting to be discovered when you are ready to accept it.

❍ When you feel that you are complete with your experience, begin conscious breathing.

Notes

Notes

- Check in with yourself. Is there something else that you need to do to feel complete? If you need something else, try **Gratitude** on your heart again, and rub three times clockwise. The vibration of *thank you* is a higher place of consciousness. It draws us to a profound state of being that helps us to attain that which we desire.

- Once again, when you feel that you are complete with the meditative experience, begin conscious breathing. Lightly cup your hands over your nose and mouth so that you have the opportunity to inhale the oils that are on your hands. This is the way to get the most benefit. Slowly come back to reality.

Trust the process and begin to listen to that inner voice within you! Daily practice of this or other kinds of meditation is a wonderful opportunity to learn ways to shift your consciousness, sharpen your intuitive skills, and to trust your Guides and Spirits. With the help of one of your favorite essential oils, you can tune into this higher consciousness at any time and on a moment's notice. You do not need a formal meditative session to do this.

The more you use your intuition, the more highly tuned it will become. The more you connect to your Spirit Guides, the easier it is to do. There is an immense amount of self-respect and pleasure, as well as spiritual and emotional balance that comes from your connection to your Higher Source.

Method 2

Connecting to Your Sacred Space

For when I don't have time to meditate, I created this technique to connect to my spiritual inner space, my place of inner being. You can use this simple and effective procedure with only a few quiet moments. A friend of mine sits at her desk before she goes into big meetings and sets her intentions this way. I find it helpful for me as a prelude to a day of giving massage or for centering before each class that I teach.

Notes

Auricular Chakras

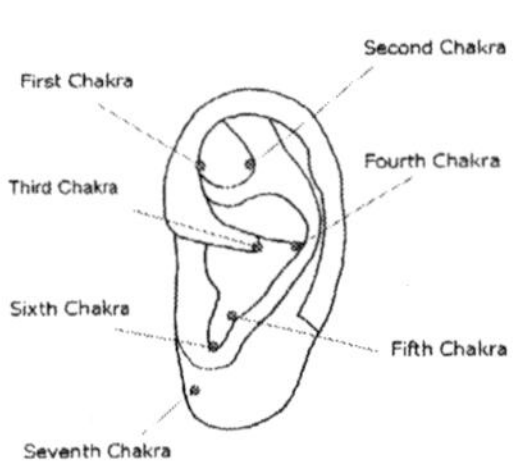

Sea of Tranquility

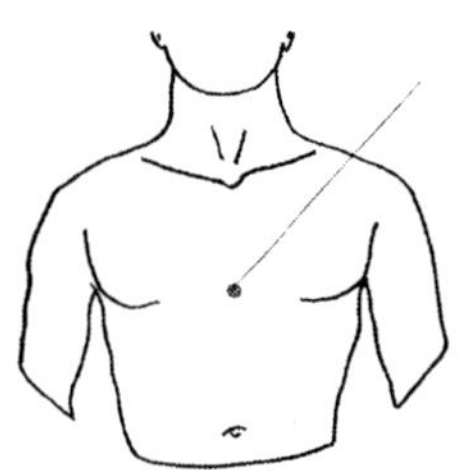

- Apply **Inspiration** on the ears, especially to the chakra points. I like to cover my entire ears, giving myself a mini ear massage.
- Place **3 Wise Men** on the Crown chakra.
- Apply **Joy** over the heart area at the acupressure point called the *Sea of Tranquility.* This point is located on the center of the sternum (breastbone), three thumb widths up from the base of the bone. You will know when you have located it because it will be slightly tender to the touch. According to acupressure theory, the *Sea of Tranquility* point may help to relieve nervousness, anxiety, chest tension and other emotional imbalances, thus reducing the effects of stress and restoring a sense of calm.
- Using your right hand, lightly place the middle fingertip directly on the *Sea of Tranquility* point and allow your index and ring fingertips to rest gently just above and below the middle finger. Breathe slowly and gently. Continue to hold your fingertips here while you progress to the next step.
- With your left hand, place the tip of your middle finger lightly on your crown. Again, your index and ring fingertips may rest slightly on either side of your middle finger.

- Continue breathing slowly and gently with focus on your breathing. Be aware of your calmer state of being. Now, verbalize your intentions and your affirmations.

- Affirmations might include the following:

    - I am the guardian of my soul.
    - There is only one person responsible for me and that is me.
    - I come from my self-esteem, not from my ego.
    - My emotional happiness is a function of my own doing. No other person, object, or situation causes anything other than the state of being that I choose.
    - There is only one me, and there is only one person who can make decisions for me.
    - It is my job to take care of me in this lifetime because I come first.
    - My soul incarnated into this body, and my soul did this for some very specific lessons that, before coming here, I chose to learn. Therefore, it is my job to accept and acknowledge the lessons, thus adding to my conscious awareness.
    - There is only one me. I am the only one who can change my life circumstance.
    - I am loved. The source of love is infinite.

Notes

Notes

- When you feel that you are complete with this experience, begin conscious breathing. Lightly cup your hands over your nose and mouth so that you have the opportunity to inhale the oils that are on your hands. Slowly come back to reality.

I use this technique frequently, and I experiment with the oils that I use. It is great for reducing stress at work or even helping me to get to sleep at night—use it any time you need a gentle reminder to restore calm.

Method 3

Regain Your Power with Present Time

We all lead busy lives. We have goals, connections, commuting schedules, meetings, social commitments, and the kids' sports practice, all with timeframes and deadlines. And then we have our cell phones, Blackberrys, and iPods to keep the mind chatter going even if we do have a free moment to ourselves.

This lack of free time assures the ego's dominance as we operate exclusively through the mind and project that same way of thinking into the future. We treat the present time as though it is an enemy, a place to escape from, and propel ourselves into the future in an attempt to escape the past. This reinforces our emotional patterns based on our past experiences.

Most of us spend our waking moments either obsessed with the past or concerned about the future, because the past holds our identity and the future embraces our opportunity for completeness. We want the emotions of dissatisfaction from the past to change into feelings of fulfillment in the future. The bridge between the past and the future is the present time, which is the place where we do our emotional healing and spiritual connecting.

We need time for being totally present with ourselves—being in the *Now*, being for the sake of understanding our beingness. I created these Present Time Exercises because I believe that being in present time is so important.

We live in the now. Every moment of every day is always the present moment, but the ego would really rather be anywhere else than in the present, because in the present we are in reality.

I once saw a person in a yoga studio wearing a t-shirt that said, "Meditation. It's not what you think." I did not found out where they got the t-shirt, but I never forgot the message. Ego coerces us into identifying with our thoughts, and so the concept around not thinking and being present during meditation is a foreign concept to most people. Present time is the space, the inner silence, when we quiet the mind and tune into our consciousness, expanding into our inner beingness.

The essential oil blend of **Present Time** is wonderful to create the energy around this state of being.

Here is an exercise that I use to help me get tuned into my inner silence.

- Apply **Grounding** or **Australian Blue** to *Bubbling Spring* on the bottoms of the feet.

- Apply **Inner Child** or **Forgiveness** clockwise around your navel three times. Next apply the oil to the *Point Zero* auricular point on your ears, pressing gently but firmly with your index finger for 30 seconds. *Point Zero* is the auricular correspondent of the umbilical cord. The navel, and reflectively *Point Zero*, is considered the physiological center of the body, the axis of energy, hormones, and brain activity.

- Apply **Present Time** to the thymus, located behind the sternum (breastbone) below the notch in the bone and above the heart. It is considered a master controller that regulates healing energies of the body.

- Also apply **Present Time** to the Third Eye chakra. This is the area of the pineal gland, which is involved with rhythmic daily and seasonal activities.

Notes

Bubbling Spring

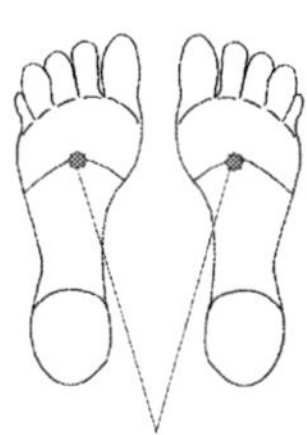

Point Zero

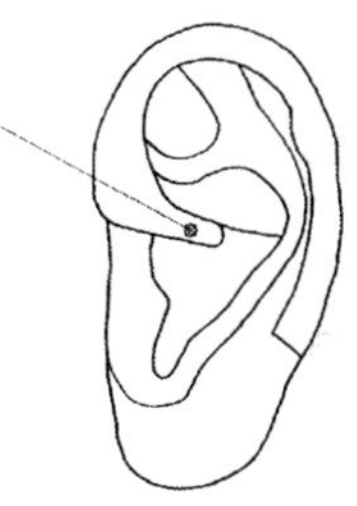

Thymus

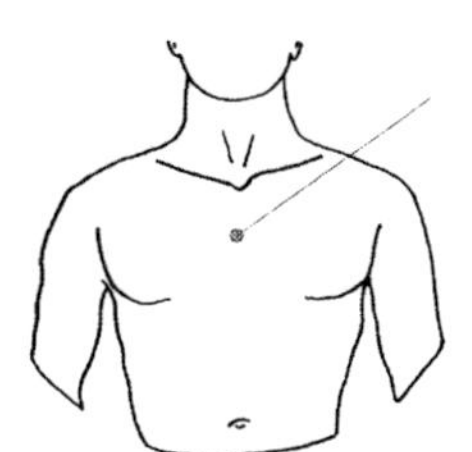

Seven Major Chakras

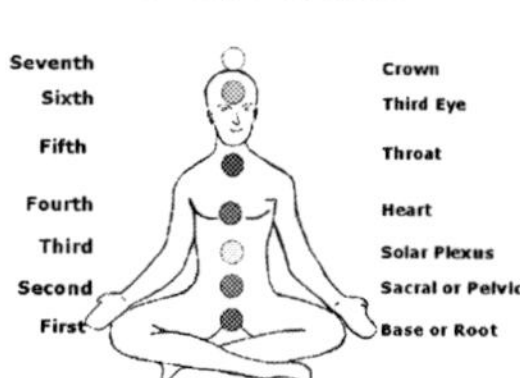

Notes

Auricular Chakras

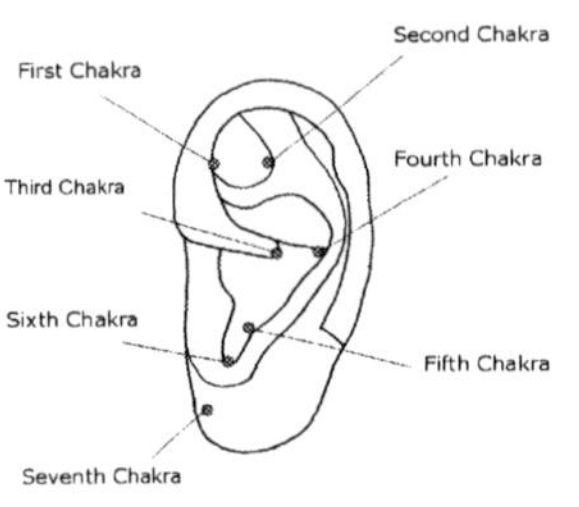

- Optionally, place **Present Time** on the auricular points for the Heart (fourth) and Third Eye (sixth) chakras.

- Continue breathing slowly and gently, focusing on your breath. Be aware of your calmer state. Now, verbalize your intentions and your affirmations.

- Affirmations might include the following:

  - My emotional hang-ups are a thing of the past. I am now in present time.

  - My future is mine to create because I am now in the present.

  - I am present with my time. My past is my past, and my future is mine to choose.

  - Today is an exciting day filled with choices. I choose to release the past and embrace the future. I choose to release my limitations and to explore my expansiveness. I choose to allow myself to be present with love and mindfulness.

  - The following affirmation, called *Being All You Can Be*, is very powerful when stated with focused intent—simply reciting it will not have the same impact. You receive the highest value of this affirmation when someone else has you repeat it after them. This helps the shift from absence of love to love energy. I modified it for consistency with the references to frequency in this book and what we know about the energy of essential oils.

Notes

<u>*Being All You Can Be*</u>[2]

"I take back my power from all to whom I have given it throughout this entire lifetime. I take my power back, NOW!

I ask to raise my cellular vibration to 75 million[3] or greater or whatever my body can handle. NOW!

(say your name), I love you. You are wonderful, magnificent and perfect as you are. And I love being you!"

- When you feel that you are complete with this experience, begin conscious breathing. Lightly cup your hands over your nose and mouth so that you have the opportunity to inhale the oils that are on your hands. Slowly come back to reality.

A surprising benefit for me in practicing the Present Time Exercises is that I have increased memory recall, especially for remembering people's names. This concept of name recall has always been difficult for me and has been the nemesis for many people I know. I have studied memory programs where you try to associate an image or a clue to remember someone's name, but these techniques did not work for me. Being in the present moment has begun to make a definite shift in my ability to recall names and faces.

---

[2] With permission from Hank Innerfeld
[3] 75 MHz

Notes

Present time means being in the now—recognizing the humanness of your spiritual being, not someone's father or mother, not someone's brother or sister, and not a friend of someone in need. Just who you are, and the specialness of you here on earth, with your needs, wants, and planetary aspects that govern and direct you toward personal self-actualization.

Method 4

Healing Bath Ritual

I learned this "Ritual Clearing Bath" technique[4] at massage school. Over time, I have modified it, emphasizing the use of essential oils as an integral part of the experience. Once again, adding essential oils to any healing modality strengthens the outcome by allowing the physical body to shift, the emotional body to release unwanted patterns, and the spiritual soul to awaken from within.

I love this technique because you can adapt the ritual to facilitate the release of any emotions that are bothering you. It is particularly helpful for those who have past issues of abuse or feelings of being used. Initially, I found it valuable to let go of past emotional programming associated with relationships. Other times, it can be helpful to re-center around a particular situation.

You can intuitively modify it to suit your needs. For the first time, follow the routine as described below.

[4] With permission from Judith Mangus

Notes

For subsequent bath ritual experiences, allow your intuition to guide your emotional healing.

Start by connecting to your sacred space and assuring yourself that you are in present time, follow the exercises in Method 2: *Connecting to Your Sacred Space* and Method 3: *Regain Your Power with Present Time*.

Bath Ingredients

- 4 oz Dead Sea Salt or Himalayan Crystal Salt
- 10 drops of your favorite essential oil, oil blend, or your customized formula (see ideas below)
- 12 oz Epsom Salt

Other Preparations

- A white candle
- Your list of intentions that you wish to release
- A bath cushion for your head (optional)
- Sacred, private space to speak out loud, cry, or whatever is needed
- Sufficient time so as not to be interrupted

Prepare your bath salts. In a ceramic cup or glass, stir the essential oils into the Dead Sea Salt or Himalayan Crystal Salt.

Add the Dead Sea Salt or Himalayan Crystal Salt and the Epsom Salt to the water as your bath is filling. Mix the bath fairly warm, as you will be in there awhile. Make sure that there is enough reserve hot water for rinsing and washing your hair afterward.

Notes

Have **Forgiveness, Release,** and **Grounding** easily accessible to you, in case you need to inhale or apply these oils during the procedure. You will be using **Gratitude** at the end.

Based on your intentions, you will call in each person who has hurt you. During this exercise, speak out loud so you can hear your voice. Hearing the spoken word reinforces the message to the conscious mind.

When ready to enter the bath, light the candle while setting the goal of releasing and healing your emotional wounds.

Begin the Experience

- Once in the bath, begin conscious breathing. Allow the flow of the Universe, your Higher Source, and the Guides or Angels that you might call on to assist you in this process. Let your breath be regular and steady, but remain conscious of it flowing in and out of your body. Feel it to the tips of your fingers and the ends of your toes. Focus on the aroma coming from the essential oils in the water; inhale the scent into every fiber of your being.
- Call in the energy of the person you wish to address.
- Forgive them for any hurt they have caused you.

Notes

- Forgive yourself for anything you did to hurt them or contribute to the situation.
- Release any and all energy of theirs that you are carrying with you, as it does not serve your highest good.
- Thank them for the lessons of growth.
- Release them and wish them well.
- Pause for conscious breathing. Go on to the next person and repeat the six steps above.
- After all have been released, pull the plug and watch the water drain as you visualize all pain and hurt going down the drain.
- When the bath is empty, take a shower and wash you hair with the intention of releasing any left over energy so that you feel complete.
- Dry yourself off with love and gratitude for your healing. Place **Gratitude** over your heart. The vibration of *thank you* is a higher place of consciousness. It draws us to a profound state of being that helps us to attain that which we desire.
- Blow out the candle with the same intention.

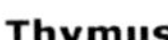

Thymus

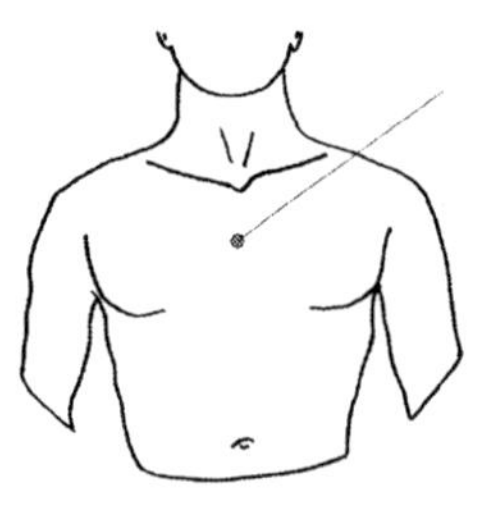

From here, I apply **Present Time** on the thymus point and repeat some of the affirmations from Method 3: *Regain Your Power with Present Time* to help me stay focused. I especially like to say the *Being All You Can Be* affirmation, repeated here for convenience.

- Affirmations might include the following:

Notes

- My emotional hang-ups are a thing of the past. I am now in present time.
- My future is mine to create because I am now in the present.
- I am present with my time. My past is my past, and my future is mine to choose.
- Today is an exciting day filled with choices. I choose to release the past and embrace the future. I choose to release my limitations and to explore my expansiveness. I choose to allow myself to be present with love and mindfulness.
- The following affirmation called *Being All You Can Be* is very powerful when stated with focused intent—simply reciting it will not have the same impact. You receive the highest value of this affirmation when someone else has you repeat it after them. This helps the shift from absence of love to love energy. I modified it for consistency with the references to frequency in this book and what we know about the energy of essential oils.

Being All You Can Be

"I take back my power from all to whom I have given it throughout this entire lifetime. I take my power back, NOW!

I ask to raise my cellular vibration to 75 million or greater or whatever my body can handle. NOW!

Notes

(say your name), I love you. You are wonderful, magnificent and perfect as you are. And I love being you!"

Sample Personalized Oil Blends

At a recent aromatherapy class, I asked the massage school students to create their own blends for this healing bath ritual. Here are some that they came up with:

Cistus and **Cedarwood**

Lavender, **Rosemary**, **Cedarwood**, and **Rosewood**

Cistus and **Believe**

Idaho Balsam Fir, Frankincense, Rosewood, and **Rosemary**

Creating a Gift for Others

For those who are important to you, prepare the 4 ounces of Dead Sea Salt or Himalayan Crystal Salt mixed with essential oil to give as gifts. Accompany your gift with copies of this bath ritual. The salt and oil combinations will stay fresh for about six months.

Dead Sea Salt can be ordered from www.seasalts.com. Himalayan Crystal Salt is available through www.americanbluegreen.com.

Method 5

Essential Oils for Your Highest Good

This has become one of my favorite routines because it helps me set my spiritual and mental tuning for the day. Instead of guessing which oils would be of help or relying on my logical brain to figure that out, I connect to my Higher Source to customize an essential oil program specifically designed for me. The program is based on setting my intentions for the day and then choosing essential oils to magnify those intentions for my highest good. This eliminates guesswork and relieves the boredom of repeatedly using the same oils.

Every day is different because the Universal Life Force energies shift and change, and my human existence needs re-alignment. My intentions

Notes

for today are not the same as those of yesterday or tomorrow.

Why not give my spiritual and emotional being the best of what is available by taking time each day to customize a program to support my best intentions? I use a pendulum and dowse to get the information available to me on an unconscious level. Muscle testing is also an option, and the concepts work the same way for these techniques.

Both techniques, muscle testing and dowsing, require that you ask questions that have a yes or no answer or a specific numeric response. With a set of procedures that answer these questions, you are able to select those oils that best serve your intentions for your greatest purpose and for those interacting with you. (For more information on muscle testing and dowsing, visit the website www.aromatherapyforthesoul.com.)

The three-step process requires that you (1) find out how many oils you need to enhance the outcome of your intention, (2) determine which oils to use, and (3) learn the sequence or order in which you should apply the oils.

- Line the bottles of oils up in rows. This facilitates the use of the pendulum or muscle testing as you check each row for the oils that you will use based on the response to the questions that you ask. My personal preference is to place the oils in alphabetical order because I can pull an oil from the row and replace it again in the same spot.

Notes

- Start by setting your intention for the day. Then ask, "Based on my intention of (*state your intention)*, how many essential oils do I need for my highest good today?" You may choose to adapt this sentence for a specific purpose. For example, you might modify it to say, "How many essential oils do I need to apply...

  ...for creating an atmosphere of faith and confidence in my abilities?"

  ...for giving me the courage to make that presentation?"

  ...for helping me to face the challenges that lie ahead?"

- From dowsing or muscle testing, the "How many essential oils do I need?" question will return a number, generally in the range of four to six. This will be the quantity of oils that you are searching for.

- Now, dowse or muscle test row by row, and ask, "Are there any oils in this row that I need?" If you get a *no,* then proceed to the next row in sequence. If the response is *yes,* then begin checking the individual oil bottles in that row for the one(s) indicated using the question, "Is this one of the oils that I need?" To speed up the process, I sometimes work in groups of three and ask, "Is the oil I need in this group of three?" When the oil is identified, pull it from the row and set it aside.

- Once a bottle is selected from a row, use this question to speed up the process, "Are there any more oils in this row?"

Notes

- After you have selected the pre-determined number of oils, ask again if there are any more oils that you should use. Use the question, "Are there any other oils here that I need for (*re-state your intention*)?" If you get a *yes* indication, go back and check again; otherwise, you are finished with this step.

- Gather the oils that you have set aside and line them up about an inch apart in a row in front of you. This time, you will be asking for the sequence or order in which you should apply them. Start with the following question, "Please show me the first oil to apply." Allow the pendulum to swing. The direction of the pendulum points to the oil bottle that answers your question. To keep track of the oils in the order indicated by this testing, pull that oil bottle from the group and start a new column of oils. Then for each of the succeeding oils, use the same technique, asking, "What is the next oil?" Line the bottles up in the new order.

If you are muscle testing, the process is similar. For all oils in the row, you would test for strong or weak to the question, "Is this the first oil that I should use?" Once the first oil is selected, continue through the remaining oils with the follow-up question, "Is this the next oil that I should use?" until you have the oils lined up in the order that you will use them.

Notes

- Apply the oils in the sequence you just determined. Looking up a specific oil or oil blend in the *Essential Oils Desk Reference* (published by Essential Science Publishing) is helpful for instructions as to where to apply the oil or the specific benefits and uses of the oils. Once you know the specific benefits, you might draw your own conclusion as to where to apply it.

For example, here are some of my intentions and the oils that were chosen by this process. I have also included the location where I applied the oils.

Intention: To have a highly successful day.

Oils and Location:

Abundance – second chakra, Sacral or Pelvic

Inspiration – Crown, Third Eye, occiput, temples

Frankincense – ear massage

Acceptance – Heart

Gratitude – Solar Plexus

Notes

Intention: To strengthen and support me mentally, emotionally, and spiritually

Oils and Location:

Idaho Balsam Fir – occiput (base of skull)

Awaken – chakras, auricular chakras

Humility – behind ears, carotid arteries (sides of neck)

Egyptian Gold – wrists

White Angelica – tops of shoulders, sternum, back of neck

Intention: To have clarity and ease in making all of the changes to this manuscript

Oils and Location:

Tangerine – back of neck

Coriander – 3 drops internal (in a capsule)

Evergreen Essence – ear massage

Rosemary – 3 drops internal (in a capsule)

3 Wise Men – chakras 1 and 7, Base and Crown

Australian Blue – chakras 3 and 5, Solar Plexus and Throat

Clarity – chakras 2 and 6, Sacral or Pelvic and Third Eye

Believe – back of neck

Gratitude – fourth chakra, Heart, and *Sea of Tranquility*

Intention: To successfully finish this book

Notes

Oils and location:

Clarity – chakras 6 and 2, Third Eye and Sacral or Pelvic

Forgiveness - clockwise around navel

3 Wise Men – chakras 1 and 7, Base and Crown, ear chakras

Present Time – thymus

Gathering - fourth chakra, Heart, and *Sea of Tranquility*

Transformation – *Point Zero*

I have found this technique to have amazing benefits as I tune into my day. I seemingly glide over the rough spots, and I gain daily cumulative spiritual awakening, which stimulates self-esteem and emotional growth. This method has opened many new vistas for me by helping me to release that outward, striving, stressful energy and to know and value my peaceful inner sanctum.

Method 6

Emotional Clearing

Emotional Clearing Technique

The ancient Egyptians practiced a ritual called Cleansing the Flesh and Blood of Evil Deities. Today we would call it emotional clearing or releasing emotions and memory trauma. The Ancient Egyptians sought the favor of their gods by going through this cleansing ritual with essential oils. They believed that, in order to progress into the spirit realm after death, it was necessary to free the body and mind from negative influences before dying.

Many people find that they are unable to progress in life and achieve sought-after goals and dreams due to trauma from emotional and physical abuse. Unless these deep-seated emotional issues are faced and neutralized, they can undermine ones successes, both in the present and in the future. This technique, combined with the selection of oil blends, has allowed numerous people to be liberated from emotional bondage and live life with a new-found purpose, optimism, and joy.

The oil blends in this method are inspired by ancient Egyptian cleansing rituals and help to release past trauma, reconnect with yourself, and envision the future you desire.

This method is one of many developed by D. Gary Young for the purpose of cleansing our bodies, our minds, and our spirits. People have been using Dr. Young's emotional clearing techniques for many years with great success. The *Feelings Kit* sold by Young Living Essential Oils contains six of the twelve oils presented in this exercise.

I include this technique because of my own experiences in using it and the remarkable personal growth that I have noticed as a result. I have used this procedure over 150 times, both for myself and many of my massage clients in a facilitated session. My personal embellishments—musings, affirmations, and techniques—may be found in italics after each oil description.

The method as presented here is a guide or template that is subject to your intuition. For example, if an oil does not feel right to you, please skip it and go to the next one. If you feel like introducing another single oil or blend, please do that also. If you are drawn to place the oils somewhere other than the indicated location, trust your feelings.

This technique helps you to access the place in the unconscious mind that knows so much more than the conscious mind. Give in to your inner blueprint as you use this procedure and allow for anything and everything to evolve in its own way.

You just might have an emotional release as you practice this exercise, so have a box of tissues close at hand. If you do have an emotional release, let it flow, let it flow, let it flow! When the emotional release feels complete, pick up with the order of the oils where you left off. If that seems impossible, please consider applying the oil blends of **Grounding**, **Hope,** and **White Angelica** on the areas specified.

Allow at least an hour, as you will be applying a sequence of twelve oils, giving yourself time to meditate between the application of each oil. I start my mini-meditations by feeling the energy of the oil that I just applied and focusing on the message that the oil is intended to impart. The message is in the name of the oil blend, for example, **Harmony, Forgiveness,** or **Joy.**

When I have been pressed for time, I have completed this exercise in as little as thirty minutes. In these cases, rather than meditate, I breathe deeply between each oil application and feel it benefitting me on every level. As I do this, I cup my hands lightly over my nose and mouth and inhale the oil on my hands, while imagining my breath reaching every cell with the healing aroma.

There are several preparations to consider as you set the stage for your emotional clearing. To begin, eliminate distractions by turning off phones and interruptive devices. Be sure that you are in a comfortable place. When I use this method, I like to sit in the lotus position, perhaps with a pillow elevating me under the buttocks. I sit on the floor at the edge of a coffee table or with a chair placed in front of me. The oils are lined up in order and the instructions placed either on the table or on the floor so that I can read them as I go along. I have found that it does not distract me to look at the instructions for the next oil, what it is for, and where to apply it. Once I had gotten used to the order, I typed up a simplified, streamlined sheet for easy reference. You will find that sheet at the end of this section. Please feel free to copy it.

I also like to diffuse the **Harmony** oil blend as I go through this clearing because it helps to release those stored up emotions and dissipates pent up trauma. And as I inhale deeply, I think of the **Harmony** balancing my chakras from the inside out.

Many people have asked, "How often can I do this technique?" Initially, I was doing this exercise on a very regular basis—every day for the first two weeks, then every week. I still do an emotional clearing using this method, but only as needed. The cumulative effects of this emotional clearing are positive, far reaching, and long lasting. I have used it up to three times a day over several consecutive days. Yes, that's right! Granted, I was very mellow after the third application and saw life in general and the future much differently after that!

Notes

If you really want to change your life, try using this technique or the *Feelings Kit* sold by Young Living Essential Oils twice a day, morning and night, for 30 days.

Once again, for each oil, place the drops of oil in your non-dominant hand and using your dominant hand rub in a clockwise motion three times to energize the oil. Then apply the oil to the place on your body as specified, or where you are directed by your intuition.

- **Valor** helps balance body energies, encouraging feelings of confidence and self-esteem.

  Sit on the floor with your knees bent and the bottoms of your feet facing each other. Place three to six drops of **Valor** in your left hand. Using the fingertips of your right hand, stir the oil clockwise three times to energize the oil. Apply the oil to the bottom of your right foot. Repeat the process with the left foot. Now, hold the palms of your hands on the bottom of your feet with your right hand on your right foot and your left hand on your left foot. The palm of your hand should fit snugly at the arch of your foot, allowing your fingertips to curl around the outside of your feet. After a few minutes, you will feel the energy beginning to pulsate between your hands and your feet, especially in the area of your arches. Once you sense the balance in both hands, you are ready to move to the next step.

  Focus on being whole and integrated, grounded to Mother Earth. Feel safe and se-

cure and know that no harm can come to you during this special time.

- **3 Wise Men,** through direct stimulation of the pineal gland, brings spiritual awareness and may help to release deep-seated trauma encoded in the DNA.

  Place three drops on the crown of the head, on the Third Eye, and on the tops of your shoulders.

  Know that you are intuitive. Know that you are connected to your Higher Source and that you are prepared to listen to the knowledge offered.

- **Harmony** promotes physical and emotional healing with harmonic balance. It helps you to let go of emotions from all areas of the body by balancing the energy centers. It is helpful to diffuse **Harmony** while going through any emotional work or during meditation.

  Place a couple of drops on each energy center, either directly on, or along the side of the body.

  I like to use this affirmation: "When I am in harmony with the Universe, all things are possible."

- **Forgiveness** may help discharge negative memories through the electrical frequencies of the oils found in this blend. It stimulates positive energy, and the fragrance allows us to forgive, forget, and heal.

Notes

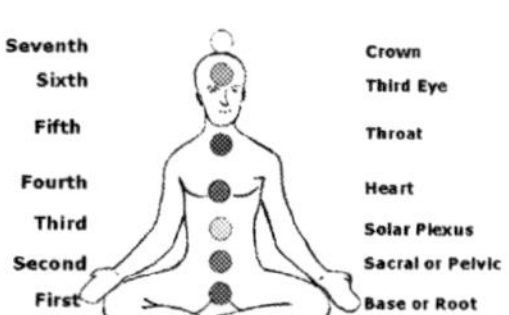

Notes

Point Zero

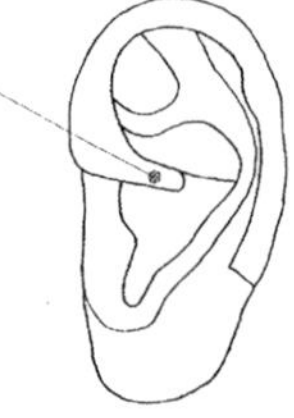

Sea of Tranquility

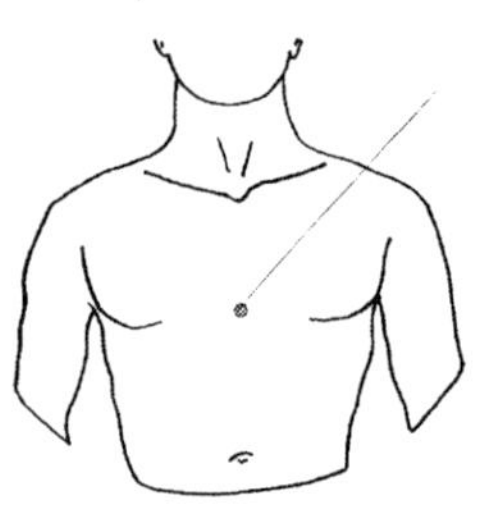

Apply with the right hand clockwise around the navel.

*Place **Forgiveness** on the Point Zero auricular point. Forgiveness is a soul choice to no longer operate in a state of disharmony within your self and with others. Forgiving yourself is equally as important as forgiving others. Forgiving does not mean absolving others from the responsibility for their actions. Rather, it is an opportunity for your soul to let go of the attachment to the anguish that it has been carrying around.*

- **Joy** is an exotic, luxurious blend that produces an uplifting magnetic energy that brings joy to the heart. It exudes an alluring and irresistible fragrance, inspiring romance and togetherness.

Apply **Joy** over the heart area.

Include the acupressure point called the Sea of Tranquility. This point is located on the center of the sternum (breastbone), three thumb widths up from the base of the bone. You will know when you have located it because it will be slightly tender to the touch. According to acupressure theory, the Sea of Tranquility point may help to relieve nervousness, anxiety, chest tension, and other emotional imbalances, thus reducing the effects of stress and restoring a sense of calm.

Lightly place the tips of the fingers of your right hand on the Sea of Tranquility point and the tips of the fingers of your left hand on your crown. In polarity theory, this forms a connection between your head and your heart, permitting synergistic balance. Imagine your heart linked to the Universal energy coming in through the crown of your head. Relax and breathe, feel your head and heart unite in peace and joy.

Notes

- **Present Time** has an empowering fragrance that engenders a feeling of being in the moment. One can only go forward and progress when one is in the present. (See also the exercise, *Regain Your Power with Present Time.*)

  Apply the oil clockwise over the thymus, located behind the sternum (breastbone), approximately 1½ inches below the notch in the bone and above the heart. After applying the oil, tap the thymus and say out loud "present time" or "in the now" three times. Use a rhythmic motion as you tap; for example, "present time" would be two taps, one tap for the word "present," another tap for the word "time."

Thymus

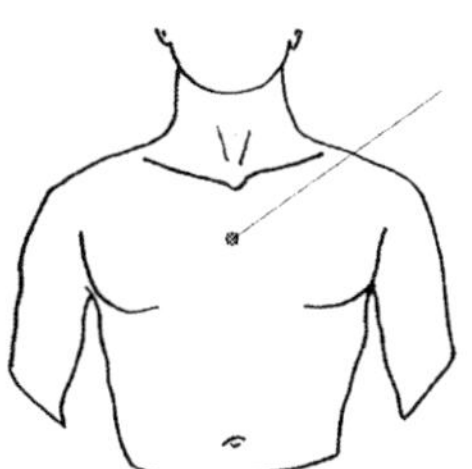

Because our emotions become sealed or ingrained through past repetitive experiences, we constantly live the present by experiencing the past. That only serves to repeat or reinforce the previous unhappy circumstances. Appreciating that we live in present time and that we have control and responsibility for our emotions and spiritual awakenings in present time opens a vast opportunity to let go of the past and embrace the future.

Notes

- **Release** may stimulate a sense of harmony and balance within the mind and body and help to let go of anger and frustration, bringing about a sense of peace and emotional well-being.

  Use three to six drops and massage gently over the liver. Allow yourself to let go. The liver is the largest gland in the body and is located under the diaphragm, more to the right side of the body. The liver lies over and almost completely covers the stomach.

  Allow yourself to let go. Place your right hand on your liver and the fingers of your left hand on your crown. Hold and allow the emotional tension to dissipate. As with ***Forgiveness,*** *let go from the soul.*

- **Inner Child** is an oil blend for those who have been abused and misused. They have a tendency to be disconnected from their inner child, or identity, causing confusion. This blend may stimulate memory response and help you to reconnect with your identity, one of the first steps to finding emotional balance.

  Tune into your Higher Source and ask for directions as to where to apply this oil, and do as you are directed. You may wish to place it around the navel, the heart, on the sternum, on the throat, behind the ears, on the temples, or on the nose.

  Put a drop of oil on the pad of your thumb and then suck your thumb. The oil permeates through the palate, reaches the nasal passageway, and stimulates the organs of the emotional brain in the space above the roof of your mouth. Feel the release.

Notes

My affirmation here is, "I love myself, and I trust who I am because I know that I have been given only as much as I can handle."

We are all given challenges, but we are also endowed with the skills necessary to cope with our situation. Some of us have the fortitude to endure a great deal, while others are given challenges to the extent that their keen intellect or emotional breakthroughs allow them to rise above and become an example.

- **Grounding** helps stabilize and ground us so that we are able to deal with reality in a logical and peaceful manner. This keeps us anchored in the now.

  Apply on the sternum, to the brainstem at the base of the neck, and on the thoracic vertebrae, where the neck connects to the back.

  Being grounded restores our connectedness and stability. Also apply to the Bubbling Spring Point on the bottoms of the feet.

Bubbling Spring

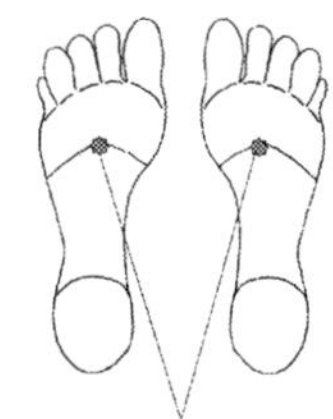

- **Hope** helps us to reconnect with a feeling of strength and grounding, restoring hope for tomorrow and helping us to go forward. It may also help to overcome severe dark thoughts, while resisting feelings of despair.

Notes

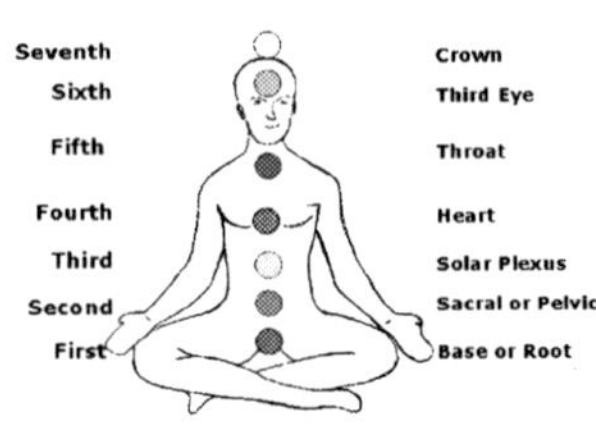

Apply to the outer rims of the ears or rub between hands and apply to the face.

My affirmation here is as follows: "I combat feelings of despair and present a new face for the future."

- **SARA** stands for *Sexual Abuse Ritual Abuse*. When inhaled, the fragrance of this oil blend facilitates the release of the traumatic memories of abuse, as well as other physical and emotional related problems. (*Note: Always use **Valor** and **Grounding** before using **SARA**.*)

  Apply over your energy centers (chakras), navel, and chest.

  When I first used this oil, it sent me into a tailspin, a way-over-the-top catharsis. Now I love the fragrance. Choose to accept and let go of all of those formidable responses to your past issues, and allow the future to open as a bright and sun-shiny place.

- **White Angelica** is a blend of oils used to increase the aura around the body, offering a delicate sense of strength and protection and a feeling of wholeness in the realm of ones own spirituality. It protects and balances the energy field.

  Apply on the tops of your shoulders, the sternum, and the back of your neck. Think of these four points as a cross.

  *I think of **White Angelica** as invoking my Guardian Angels. They are always with me,* *but this gives me an opportunity to feel their strength and commitment to me. I thank them for their protection and guardianship.*

Notes

Closing

This is the completion of the emotional clearing. At this time, I do three things. I sweep my aura to eliminate any unwanted leftover energy that remains, I verbalize an affirmation, and I do conscious breathing.

- **Sweep Your Aura:** Your energy field extends out approximately eight to twelve inches from your body. Start about fifteen inches above the seventh, or Crown chakra, and move in flowing strokes toward the feet, front to back, side to side. Your fingers should be spread slightly apart, wrists flexible. Move your hands as though you are lightly raking through your energy field. Perform long smooth motions eight to twelve inches away from the body, sweeping through your field. Start at your crown and continue to sweep out through your feet, allowing any excess energy to be absorbed by the ground. For some of you, this might seem silly. However, it is symbolic. For others who are more sensitive, you may feel areas of blockages that need additional opening, and you should continue to sweep or rake those areas until clear.
- **Affirmation:** As you sweep your energy field or just after you have finished, say this affirmation out loud:

Notes

> "I lovingly and willingly release and let go of all those things that no longer serve me. I release these things to the Universe from whence they came to be re-polarized to be a positive and progressive power for me and others. NOW."

When you feel that you are complete with this experience, begin conscious breathing. Lightly cup your hands over your nose so that you have the opportunity to inhale the oils that are on your hands. Slowly come back to reality.

Emotional Clearing Quick Summary

Directions: Photocopy this handy reference and use for emotional clearing. The locations to apply the oils are underlined for quick reference. Extra spacing is provided between each oil description for adding your own favorite technique or affirmation.

Valor - Six drops for each foot. Balance your energies by applying your hands to the soles of your feet.

3 Wise Men – Three drops on the crown of your head, Third Eye, and shoulders. Connect to your Higher Source, your spiritual awareness.

Harmony - One drop on each energy center. Let go of emotions from all areas of your body by conscious breathing and balancing the chakras.

Forgiveness - With your right hand, apply clockwise around your navel. Creates the frequency and fragrance to allow you to forgive, forget, and heal.

Joy - Rub over heart at the *Sea of Tranquility* point. Place fingertips of right hand on *Sea of Tranquility* and fingertips of left hand on crown. Connect in peace and joy.

Present Time - Massage clockwise over the thymus to regulate the body's healing energies. Rhythmically tap the thymus and say "present time" or "in the now."

Release – Massage 3-6 drops gently over liver. Allow yourself to let go.

Inner Child – Ask for directions from your Higher Source for where to apply this oil. Suggested areas are around the navel or heart, on the sternum, on the throat, behind the ears, on the temples, or on the nose. Put a drop of oil on the pad of your thumb and then suck your thumb so that the oil is absorbed through the roof of your mouth.

Grounding – One drop on the thoracic vertebrae where the neck attaches to the back at base of the neck, brainstem, sternum, and the *Bubbling Spring* point on the bottoms of the feet.

Hope - Rub on the outer rims of the ears or rub between hands and apply to face. Combats feelings of despair and presents a new face for the future.

SARA - Apply over chakras, navel, and chest. This oil enables memory trauma release. (Note: Always use **Valor** and **Grounding** before using **SARA**.)

White Angelica – Place on the tops of your shoulders, the sternum, and the back of your neck. Think of these four points as a cross. Invoke your Guardian Angels.

Sweep Your Aura – Head to toes, front to back, side to side.

Affirmation to use at the end: "I lovingly and willingly release and let go of all those things that no longer serve me. I release these things to the Universe from whence they came to be re-polarized to be a positive and progressive power for me and others. NOW."

Conscious Breathing – Lightly cup your hands over your nose; inhale the oils while breathing.

Emotional Clearing Testimonial

This testimonial comes from Artemis in Australia and I was compelled to share it in this book because it demonstrates the emotional clearing power of essential oils. In this case, Artemis used her version, which she calls the Egyptian Emotional Clearing Technique, on a horse.

I was so impressed with this testimonial because of the horse's immediate response to the application of the essential oils. Animals do not have belief systems as humans do, so they do not pre-judge a modality. They act and respond instinctively.

Egyptian Emotional Clearing Technique on Sheba the Mare

It is with great joy that I share this next story about my work with oils for horses. And just so you know, our wonderful gelding, Star, was completely over his sinus infection within three weeks of applying the oils and receiving regular Raindrop sessions. The vet who was going to put him down (or perform a $4,000 operation on him and drill out his sinuses) had no explanation for Star's complete and quick recovery. But we know the secret was in the essential oils and in Star's willingness to heal.

As I had been sharing my results on Star, a colleague asked me if I would work on another horse. This mare is called Sheba, and her problem was emotional, not physical. Her long-term paddock friend and playmate (another horse) died tragically from a wound in its neck. It bled to death and lay in the paddock for two days before it was found. Since that incident, Sheba had been a different horse. She refused to go into that paddock and kept her head down all day. She stopped galloping and she stopped responding to her owner's whistles. She kept looking toward the hill where the other horse had died.

*From the moment I heard about Sheba, I knew I wanted to work with her. I've never performed the Egyptian Emotional Clearing technique on a horse before, but I saw no reason why it wouldn't work on her. I followed the technique exactly as I would on a human. First, I approached Sheba with some **geranium** oil on the palms of my hands so she would get used to the smell (and to me).*

Then I proceeded to do the Egyptian Emotional Clearing Technique on her as follows:

*Three drops of **Valor**. I applied it on each coronet band, the fur just above her back hoofs, and held for five minutes with my right hand on her right foot and with my left hand on her left foot.*

***Harmony** oil in drops up her spine. I hoped to get it on all of her chakras, as I expect that horses have chakras just like humans.*

*One drop of **3 Wise Men** placed on her crown.*

*One drop of **Present Time** rubbed on her thymus, or as close as I could guesstimate!*

*One drop of **Inner Child** massaged on her navel. Again, I said a prayer and reached under her belly and found an indentation that felt like a navel, so that's where the oil went.*

*Three drops of **Release** applied to her liver. This oil seemed to be one of her favourites, as she kept smelling and smelling it.*

*One drop of **Dream Catcher** rubbed on her forehead at her Third Eye.*

*One drop of **Hope** dabbed on the inside of each ear.*

*One drop of **Forgiveness** massaged on her navel.*

*One drop of **Joy** rubbed on her chest.*

*One drop of **SARA** placed wherever there is trauma. Honestly, I can't remember where I put it on Sheba.*

*Three drops of **White Angelica** on each shoulder.*

*Three drops of **Grounding** spread on her sternum.*

*Intuitively, I felt that I had to use several drops of **Trauma Life** on her throat. As I was applying the oil, I wondered why I was putting it on her throat, and then I remembered that her companion had died from a wound to the throat. I realized that Sheba was acting as a surrogate for her dead companion. By putting the oil on Sheba, I was also accessing the spirit of the other horse. I felt a deep connection with both horses as I did this, and I felt that this was the turning point in the session.*

By the time I finished, Sheba was a different horse. This is according to her owner, Allan Bourquin, and not just my observations. She went out into her paddock and began galloping around. He whistled for her numerous times over the next few hours, and she put her head up each time, just like she used to.

*Since that day, he has been using **Release**—her favourite oil—on her regularly. He tells me that she is her "old self," but she still looks up to the hill where her friend died. He knows that both horses are there—Sheba in the flesh, and her friend in Spirit.*

I love the way horses respond to these oils. About half way through the treatment, Sheba insisted on smelling each of the oils as we brought them over. And she didn't just smell it! She stuck her nostril over the bottle so that the top of each bottle literally disappeared up her nose! Now that's what I call "snorting" oils!

And she became very cuddly with me, leaning up against me so that we both shared a wonderful connection.

- Artemis, Australia

Epilog

We all know that just talking about making changes is easier than actually doing whatever it takes to make them happen! The routine of everyday living lures us into a state-of-mind numbness, forever dwelling on the past and hoping that the future somehow will be different.

Thinking about that and respecting my personal life challenges, I wanted to see if these techniques could make a difference in my own situation. They did.

Taking that to the next step, I felt compelled to share with others some of the truly wondrous results of applying the Young Living Essential Oils. My journey led me to so many discoveries about enhancing life's experiences.

With this information, my intentions with this book are two-fold:

- To convey a sense of empowerment, through knowledge, as a means to effect positive change for those who want to transform their lives.
- To broaden the insight for how and why we do the things we do, in order to create a new level of conscious awareness.

My premise then becomes that the most effective ways for doing that are:

- Tuning into your Higher Self, listening to your soul's wisdom (your intuition), and choosing to be in the present.
- Enhancing all of your techniques and methods with therapeutic grade essential oils to support your body, mind, and spirit, because the oils optimize result.

The many techniques included in this book provide ideas for approaching your emotional release and conscious awakening. Some of these are new; others you might have seen in another context. All have been enhanced by including my own experiences using essential oils.

The first time you try any of these methods, it is my recommendation that you follow the instructions. The cumulative benefits of using essential oils over time will increase your intuitive powers through improved listening to your Higher Source. As you become increasingly in touch with your intuition, your ability to select the best essential oil(s) for your specific situation will also expand.

As you experiment and create your own success stories, I would love to hear from you. Some of you have already experienced a spiritual awareness through the use of essential oils; others of you are just on the horizon. Perhaps you will develop your own special method. Future editions of this book will include reader testimonials and additional methods. There is so much more to be said!

What is the final message of this book? I hope that the ideas provided here help to define you on your chosen spiritual journey. After all, it is the spiritual, intertwined with the emotional journey that is important. Listen and follow your soul's guidance and wisdom. Add essential oils to your daily routine for a better understanding of who you are and who you are choosing to become. And know that the best time to begin is now!

Namaste,
Judy Jehn

Appendix

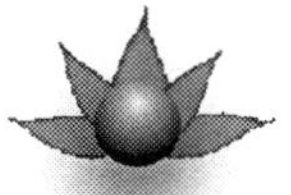

Glossary of Terms

Affirmation - An affirmation is a positive thought intended to bring about a shift in consciousness. This constructive self-talk makes a declaration or an assertion by using words in the present tense to change a pattern of thinking or an emotional awareness. An example of a general affirmation is, "Every day and in every way, things just keep getting better and better." It is suggested that you repeat affirmations over and over during the day to reinforce the thought process.

Amygdala - The amygdala gland is in the limbic area, the emotional center of the brain. The amygdala gland sits in the temporal lobe centered between the two cerebral hemispheres; it is a small almond shaped neural structure that plays a role in the sense of smell, motivation, and emotion.

Aura - This energy field around the body extends out approximately the length of your outstretched arms. The energies of the chakras overlap, with some fields being stronger than others, and this combined multitude of colors with the different wavelengths of light is known as your aura. Everyone's aura is different, and everyone's aura changes instantaneously as we interact and evolve spiritually and emotionally. This eggshell-shaped personal electromagnetic profile around each of us reflects the subtle life energies within the body. See also **Electromagnetic Field**.

Auriculotherapy - Developed in France during the mid-20th century, auriculotherapy is a modality wherein points on the external surface of the ear, or auricle, are activated to relieve conditions in other areas of the body. There are over 2,700 points of stimulation on the ear.

Blood Brain Barrier - Instead of a barrier, think of this as a sieve or filter through which only molecules of a certain size or smaller will pass through to enter the brain tissue. Lipid solubility is another factor which facilitates passage through the barrier. The molecules of essential oils are very small and lipid (fat) soluble.

Chi - The vital life force energy of the Universe is present within every living thing. The Chinese refer to the **Electromagnetic Field** or **Life Force Energy** as 'Chi' (pronounced Chee).

Chakras – The natural force fields located over specific areas in the body are called chakras. The word *chakra* comes from Sanskrit and refers to a spinning wheel. The chakras are the master coordinating centers for organizing the flow of physical, spiritual, and emotional energy, both the transmission from our bodies and the receiving into our life force.

Constituents – Essential oils are organic compounds containing mixtures of hundreds of constituents, or chemical components which are made up of carbon, hydrogen, and oxygen.

DNA – Deoxyribonucleic acid is the genetic information within the cell nucleus (the control center of the cell). It replicates itself exactly before a cell divides and it provides the instructions for building every protein in the body.

Electromagnetic Field – Everything in creation is made up of electromagnetic energy vibrating at different frequencies that correspond to sound, light, color, and smell. Science recognizes the existence of electromagnetic fields around every object in the Universe. This is known as an aura. The field of vibrating electromagnetic energy surrounding every object in the Universe is referred to as **Aura**, **Chi** (Chinese), **Ki** (Japanese), or **Prana** (Indian).

Energy Centers – see **Chakras.**

Higher Source - My reference to a *Higher Source* in this book refers to a spirituality, which I call God. You may have another name like Divinity, Spirituality, Universe, Higher Consciousness, Buddha, or whatever name that you choose.

Homeostasis – The body's ability to maintain a dynamic state of equilibrium, or internal balance, even though the outside world is constantly changing, is called homeostasis.

Immunostimulant – A substance that stimulates the immune system.

Ki – The Japanese term referring to the electromagnetic frequency surrounding the body. See also **Electromagnetic Field**.

Meridians – Within the body, Chi circulates in vertical channels, and in Traditional Chinese Medicine, these are the energy meridians of the body. There are six yin and six yang meridians always at work.

Namaste – Namaste literally means "Your humble servant," and is an expression of deep respect commonly used in India and Nepal. In yoga, namaste is said to mean "I am your humble servant," which you say to your instructor. The gesture accompanying the expression is a slight bow with the hands folded in a prayer position.

Neurotransmitter – The transmission of impulses from one nerve to the adjacent nerve occurs via a chemical or protein substance that is secreted at the synaptic membrane.

Prana – The Indian term that refers to the electromagnetic energy surrounding the body. See also **Electromagnetic Energy**.

Reiki – Reiki is the name given to a profound yet simple natural healing system for body and mind. It was developed by Dr. Mikao Usui during the 19th century in Japan. *Rei* means "universal" and *ki* means "Life Force Energy."

RNA – Ribonucleic acid is located outside the cell nucleus and carries out the orders for protein synthesis issued by the **DNA**. **RNA** is considered the slave, as it is nucleic acid that carries information from the **DNA** (the master) and translates it into a protein structural assembly within the cell.

Visualization – This is the act of seeing a picture or forming an image in your mind's eye. It is helpful to combine visualizations with **Affirmations** in a meditative experience because the modalities support each other to change the conscious reality.

Young Living Essential Oils - Young Living Essential Oils is a multinational, relationship marketing company specializing in the production and distribution of therapeutic-grade essential oils and premium products enhanced with essential oils. Young Living is the largest supplier of essential oils in the world. Young Living Essential Oils are distributed through independent representatives. For more information contact your local essential oils distributor, call Young Living directly at 800-371-2928 (#19714), or visit http://judyjehn.younglivingworld.com or www.aromamethods.com.

Precautions When Using Essential Oils

Never use water to dilute an essential oil if your skin becomes irritated or if oils get into your eyes. To dilute an essential oil, use a fat soluble substance such as vegetable oil, butter, or milk. Use milk or vegetable oil for the eyes. Water magnifies the intensity of the essential oil, while vegetable oil reduces the intensity.

Citrus oils are photosensitive and have a tendency to burn the skin if applied prior to exposure to direct sunlight, leaving a dark area on the skin for weeks. Refrain from using citrus oils on uncovered skin for two days before direct sun exposure. Only apply citrus oils to areas where the sun does not shine, the soles of the feet, behind the ears, or on the wrists.

Dilute essential oils for children. One to three drops per tablespoon of oil or milk for infants and one to three drops per teaspoon of oil for 2 to 5 year olds, and the same for pets, as a rule of thumb.

If you are pregnant, avoid the essential oils of **wintergreen**, **birch**, **lavandin**, **cumin**, **basil**, **tarragon**, **sage**, **rosemary**, **hyssop**, **savory**, and **cinnamon bark**. If you are pregnant, exercise caution in using the following oils of **peppermint**, **rose**, **vetiver**, **yarrow**, **spearmin**t, **nutmeg**, **fennel**, and **clary sage**.

If you have high blood pressure, avoid **peppermint**, **sage**, **thyme**, and **hyssop**.

Epileptics should avoid **rosemary**, **tarragon**, **hyssop**, wintergreen, **birch**, **sage**, **nutmeg**, **lavandin**, **fennel**, and **basil**.

Drink lots of water to flush out toxins being removed from the cells by the essential oils

If your skin has been exposed to chemicals such as propylene glycol, sodium laurel sulfate, or DEA, you may have a skin reaction to therapeutic grade oils, as the essential oils work to obliterate the acidity and toxins that are stored within the skin cells. Reduce (or dilute) the amount of essential oil used and cleanse (detoxify) the body of stored toxins before using essential oils full strength.

Illustrations

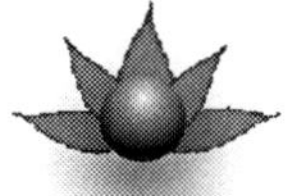

Auricular Chakras

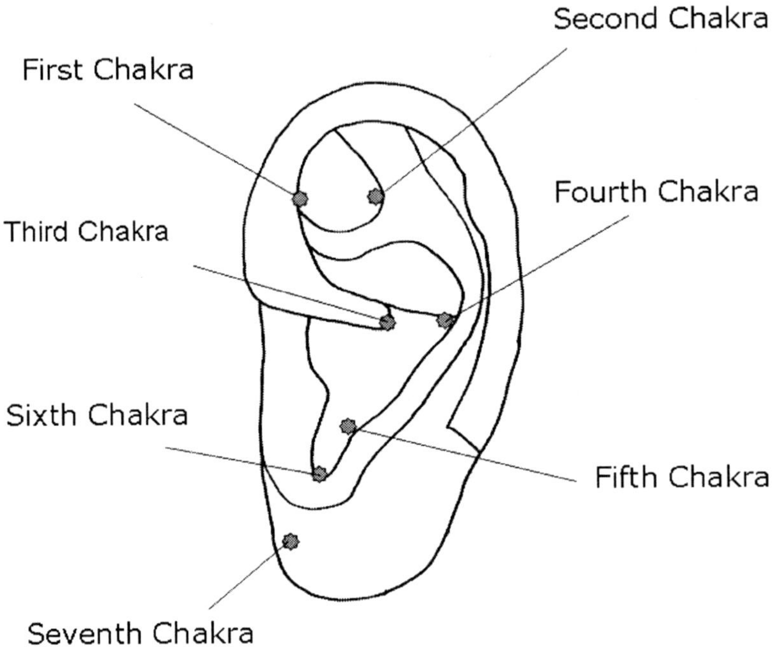

The chakras are represented on each ear. In auriculotherapy, the left ear represents the emotional body and the right ear corresponds to the physical body.

Bubbling Spring

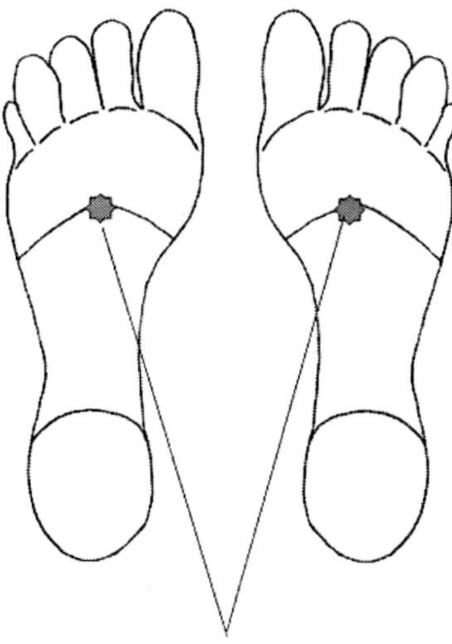

Bubbling Spring is a Chinese acupuncture point, *Kidney 1 (K 1).* It is located at the lowest energetic point in the body, on the bottom of the foot, behind the ball of the foot, in the depression in the center of the sole. It is our connection with the earth.

After applying the essential oil to *Bubbling Spring*, place your thumb on the point and alternately press and release in a pumping motion for 30 seconds to 1 minute. Repeat this press and release pumping motion on the other foot.

Chakra Life Force Energy

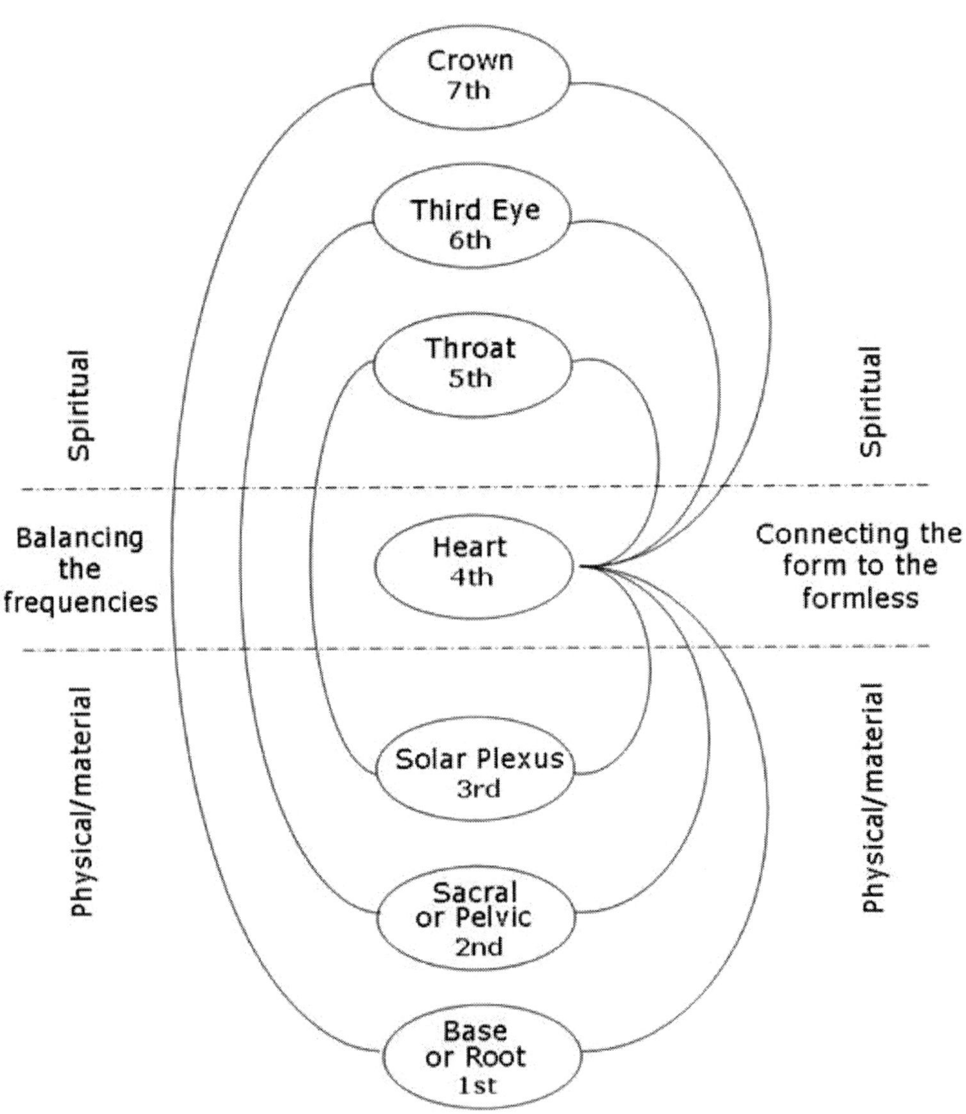

Corresponding and oppositional chakra frequencies for balance and harmonic convergence

Point Zero

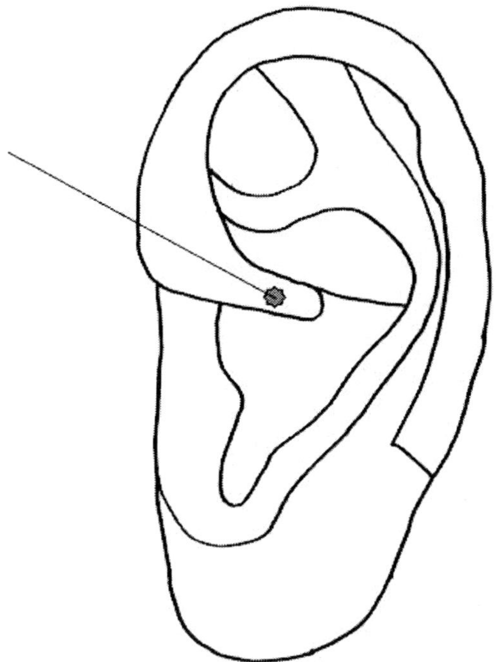

Point Zero is the auricular correspondent of the umbilical cord. The navel, and reflectively *Point Zero*, is considered the physiological center of the body, the axis of energy, hormones, and brain activity.

When applying essential oil to the *Point Zero* auricular point on your ears, press gently but firmly with your index finger for 30 seconds.

Thymus

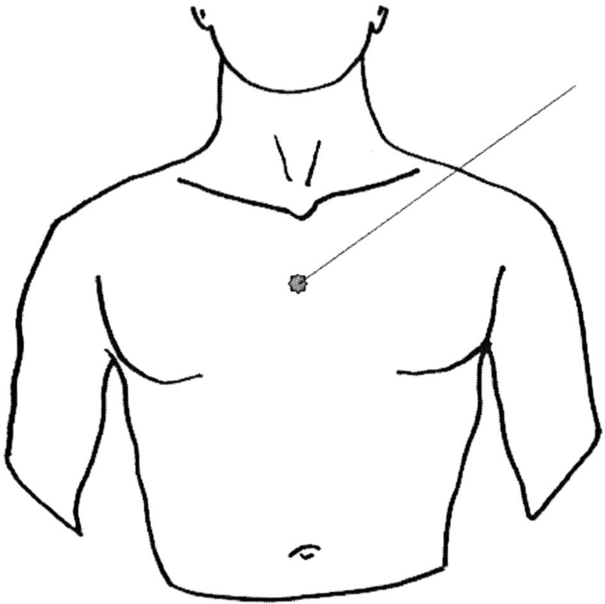

Apply **Present Time** to the thymus, located behind the sternum (breastbone) below the notch in the bone and above the heart. It is considered a master controller that regulates healing energies of the body.

Sea of Tranquility

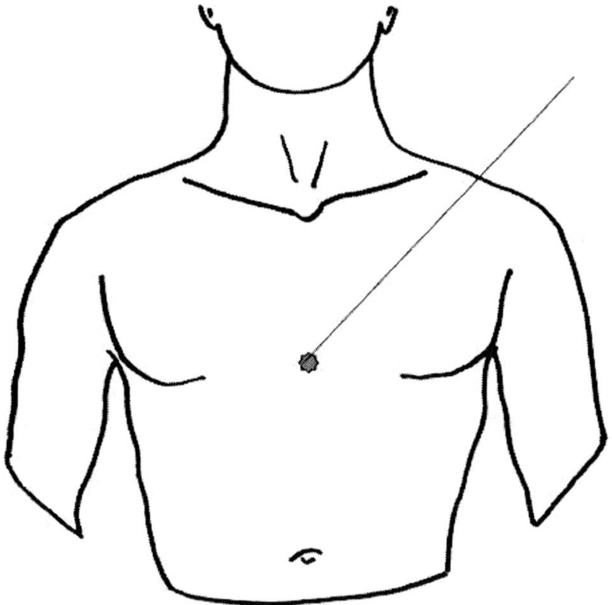

The *Sea of Tranquility* point is located on the center of the sternum, three thumb widths up from the base of the bone. You will know when you have located it because it will be slightly tender to the touch.

According to acupressure theory, the *Sea of Tranquility* point may help to relieve nervousness, anxiety, chest tension and other emotional imbalances, reducing the effects of stress and restoring a sense of calm.

Apply your favorite essential oil to this the *Sea of Tranquility* and your crown. Lightly place the fingertips of your right hand on the *Sea of Tranquility* and the fingertips of your left hand on your crown. Imagine your heart linked to the Universal energy coming in through the crown of your head. Relax and breathe, feel your head and heart unite in peace and joy.

Seven Major Chakras

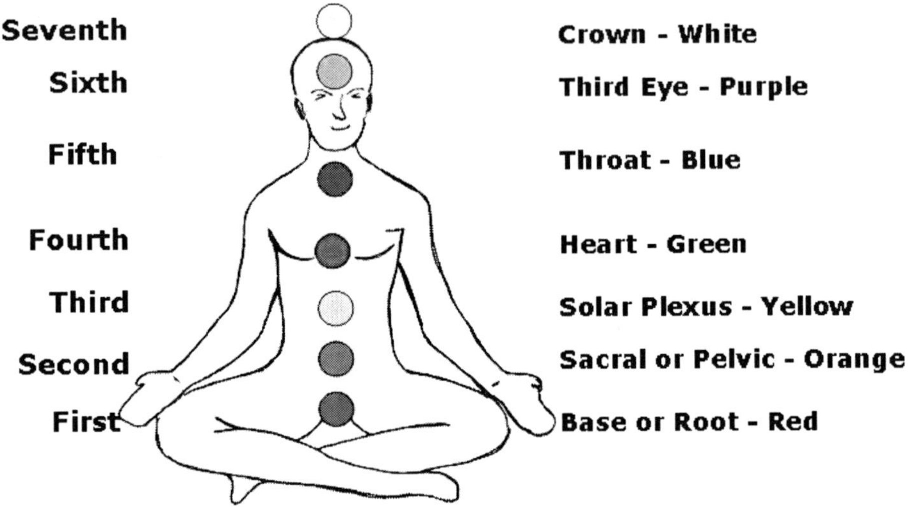

Bibliography and Webliography

Anderson, Rita M. *Nature's Hearing Aid: Essential Oils Applications for Physical and Emotional Support,* Seminar Handouts, Denver, CO, April 22, 1998

Anthony, Susie. *A Map to God: Awakening Spiritual Integrity*, O Books, Winchester, UK, and Washington, USA, 2007

Blakeslee, Sandra and Matthew. *The Body Has a Mind of Its Own: How Body Maps in Your Brain Help You Do (Almost) Everything Better, Random House, New York, NY, 2007*

Farmer, Kathy. *Unlocking Emotions with Essential Oils*, Seminar, Handout, 1997

Farmer, Kathy and Anderson, Rita. *Spiritual/Emotional Applications and Uses of Essential Oils,* Aroma Mastery Workshop Seminar, Handout, 1999

Foley, Marcy. *Embraced by the Essence: Your Journey into Wellness Using Pure Quality Essential Oils*, 2nd ed., Holistic Wellness Foundation I, Boulder, CO, 2000

Hay, Louise L. *Heal Your Body: The Mental Causes for Physical Illness and the Metaphysical Way to Overcome Them*, Hay House, Inc., Carlsbad, CA, 65th Printing, 4th ed., 2005

Holland, John. *Power of the Soul: Inside Wisdom for an Outside World,* Hay House, Carlsbad, CA, 2007

Innerfeld, Hank. *Messages to Your Heart: Insights and Understandings to Empower Your Life,* I&A Publishing, Conifer, CO, 2005

Innerfeld, Hank. Empowerment workshops, conducted various dates, 2003 to the present

Lundberg, Paul. *The Book of Shiatsu*, Simon & Schuster, Fireside, New York, NY, 2003

Mangus, Judith. *Heart Match* Class, conducted various dates

Manwaring, Brian, editor. *Essential Oils Desk Reference,* 4th ed., Essential Science Publishing, Orem, UT, 2008

Marieb, Elaine N. *Essentials of Human Anatomy & Physiology*, 7th ed., Holyoke Community College, Benjamin Cummings Pub, 2003

Mein, Carolyn L. *Releasing Emotional Patterns with Essential Oils,* 2007 ed., Vision Ware Press, Rancho Santa Fe, CA, 2007

Myss, Caroline. *Anatomy of the Spirit: The Seven Stages of Power and Healing*, Three Rivers Press, New York, NY, 1996

Myss, Caroline. *Invisible Acts of Power: Personal Choices That Create Miracles*, CD set, Sounds True, Boulder, CO, 2004

Oleson, Terry. *Auriculotherapy Manual: Chinese and Western Systems of Ear Acupuncture*, 3rd ed., Elsevier Limited, 2003

Redfield, James. *The Celestine Prophecy: An Adventure,* Warner Books, New York, NY, 1993, 2006

Russell, Ron. *Resonant Viewing*, Seminar Notes and Handouts, 2008

Sha, Zhi Gang. *Living Divine Relationships*, Elite Books, Santa Rosa, CA, 2006

Stewart, David. *Healing Oils of the Bible*, CARE Publications, Marble Hill, MO, 2003

Tolle, Eckhart. *A New Earth: Awakening to Your Life's Purpose,* A Plume Book, USA, 2006

Truman, Karol K., *Feelings Buried Alive Never Die...*, Olympus Distributing, St. George, UT, 10th Printing, 2004

Young, D. Gary. *Essential Oils Integrative Medical Guide,* Essential Science Publishing, USA, 2003

Young, D. Gary. *Aromatherapy: The Essential Beginning*, 2nd ed. Essential Science Publishing, Orem, UT, 1996

Vennells, David F. *Reiki for Beginners,* Llewellyn Publications, St. Paul, MN, 2002

Acknowledgements

I am indeed fortunate to have a wonderful group of friends and colleagues who respect and love me for being just who I am. Their confidence in me has given me the courage to continue to forge ahead. And their belief that I could and should write this book touches me to my core.

I want to express my appreciation to all of my mentors, and especially to three women who are wonderfully heart-centered, that is to say that their Heart Chakras simply radiate! Diane Mora's love glows with her generosity, both in the gracious sharing of her time and her giving nature, helping others to recognize their highest potential. Helen Grigg, RMT, with her inner strength and spiritual connectedness, has the gift of holding space for those in emotional need and the grace for encouraging them to continue through their healing process. Patricia Fleischer, RMT is a constant source of inspiration, kindness, and cheerfulness.

I wish to thank Lori Blassingame, Cindy Goral, Valena Hunley, and my mom, Betty Jehn, who offered helpful suggestions for improving the quality and clarity of this manuscript. I am especially grateful to Kathryn Caywood for her masterful editing skills, clarity, insight, and above all, her friendship and humor.

I also appreciate the time spent with Dr. Edward Sullivan D.C., Ph.D., DipL.AC; he generously shared his vast knowledge of auriculotherapy. With his help, we began the process of applying essential oils to the auricular ear points.

Most of all, I wish to thank D. Gary Young and the incredible Young Living Essential Oils for helping me to be where I am today. I owe my physical and emotional revitalization to the Young Living oils and the knowledge and generosity of Gary Young. I would also like to thank Mary Young for being a model of strength and commitment and an example of how beautiful we can be.

A portion of the proceeds of this book will be donated to the D. Gary Young Foundation. For more information on this organization, please go to www.dgaryyoungfoundation.org.

About the Author

Judy Jehn, RMT is a gifted massage therapist and an exuberant teacher. Her passion is aromatherapy. She believes that the use of therapeutic essential oils for physical, mental, emotional, and spiritual empowerment enable individuals to pro-actively embrace their health and well-being.

Judy has studied and taught aromatherapy since 1993 and the quality and depth of her seminars have impacted thousands of lives throughout the United States. Additionally, in the Denver, Colorado area, she teaches essential oil aromatherapy to nursing homes and massage therapists.

Reverend Judy Jehn practices Raindrop Therapy, Spiritual Response Therapy, Reiki, Yuen Method and therapeutic massage techniques. She is available for lectures and private appointments for massage. Judy can be reached at judy@aromatherapyforthesoul.com.

Index

S

T

U

V

Y

Printed in the United States
134468LV00007B/8/P

9 780981 829005